Otoscopy Findings

Janez Rebol

Otoscopy Findings

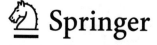

Janez Rebol
Department of Otorhinolaryngology
University Clinical Centre Maribor
Maribor, Slovenia

ISBN 978-3-031-03981-2   ISBN 978-3-031-03979-9   (eBook)
https://doi.org/10.1007/978-3-031-03979-9

This Springer imprint is published by the registered company Springer Nature Switzerland AG
The registered company address is: Gewerbestrasse 11, 6330 Cham, Switzerland

Preface

In otology, paediatrics, and general medicine, accurate diagnosis of ear diseases relies heavily on otoscopy. During my practice in the field of otology, I have been able to collect a large number of images of pathological ear conditions, which I believe can enhance the learning process in the areas mentioned above.

In otoscopy, a proper light source and a way to magnify the image are very important. Very often, proper cleaning of the ear canal is also required. Experience, hard to obtain during study years, is of great importance.

The images in this volume were collected over 15 years at the Department of Otorhinolaryngology of the Maribor University Medical Centre. A commentary accompanying each image explains the findings and the conditions that led to the disease. Diagnoses in otology are also made with the help of audiological and other examinations, but this book focuses on otoscopy.

The identification of those conditions in which surgical intervention is mandatory is especially important. With this in mind, many images of cholesteatoma, secretory otitis, and chronic otitis have been included.

The number of patients with cochlear implants (CI) and bone conduction devices (BCD) is increasing and, in view of this, images relating to CI and BCD with additional images of the major surgical procedures or conditions associated with them are included.

As well as a good otoscope, a great deal of practice with patients is also essential. Over the years I estimate that, besides ear operations, I have carried out more than 210,000 otoscopies. How many are needed to avoid the overtreatment of acute otitis media is difficult to say. I do hope, however, that this book will assist in attaining the knowledge required for successful otologic examination and treatment.

This book is aimed at medical students and residents in otolaryngology, paediatrics, and general medicine.

During my teaching and mentoring of residents, I often find that they have difficulties in explaining what they are seeing during an otoscopy and are uncertain of what to look for, thus often overlooking the pathology. They also have trouble examining children where the otoscopy has to be conducted swiftly and cannot be repeated.

The majority of otoscopic images were taken with a Storz otoscope using an electronic flash and an attached endocamera.

I hope and expect that students and residents will take this book into the clinic and compare the images presented with actual otoscopy examinations in patients. Ideally, they might also discuss their findings with their senior colleagues and mentors.

Maribor, Slovenia   Janez Rebol

Acknowledgment

I would like to thank doc. Gerhard Moser from Salzburg for reviewing the manuscript.

Contents

Otoscopy

1

Otoscopy is a routine examination for ENT specialists, general practitioners, and paediatricians and is a key step in diagnosing ear conditions. Clinical examination with the speculum otoscope is not always straightforward. It may be hindered by cerumen blockage, secretions in the external ear canal, poor luminosity, and malposition of the otoscope.

Good illumination is essential for all successful otoscopy, either using headlight investigation, an otoscope (Fig. 1.1), or a microscope (Fig. 1.3). When purchasing an otoscope, it is important to look for devices with good illumination, even though the cost might be higher. A study of otoscopes used by private practice physicians found that one third of the devices had a suboptimal output of light. One third of the physicians participating in the same study changed the otoscope bulbs less often than the recommended every 2 years, and in almost half the devices the rechargeable batteries were found to be out of date [1].

The ear can also be examined very well with a tele-otoscope with a cold light source (Fig. 1.2).

ENT specialists now mostly use the microscope, which enables bimanual working in the external ear canal and on the ear drum (Fig. 1.3).

It is estimated that reliance on the monocular otoscope to diagnose ear disease has a 50% higher chance of misdiagnosis in comparison with binocular microscopic otoscopy.

When examining the ear, we should first straighten the external ear canal (EAC) by pulling the pinna upwards and then insert the ear speculum into the EAC. To avoid injury of the EAC, it is necessary to rest either the index finger or the little finger of the hand holding the otoscope against the patient's head. In every examination position, mobility, colour, and the degree of translucency should be described and evaluated. The normal tympanic membrane is in a neutral position (neither retracted nor bulging), pearly grey, translucent, and responding to changes in air pressure. The colour of the ear drum is of lesser importance than the membrane's position and mobility [2].

© The Author(s), under exclusive license to Springer Nature
Switzerland AG 2022
J. Rebol, *Otoscopy Findings*, https://doi.org/10.1007/978-3-031-03979-9_1

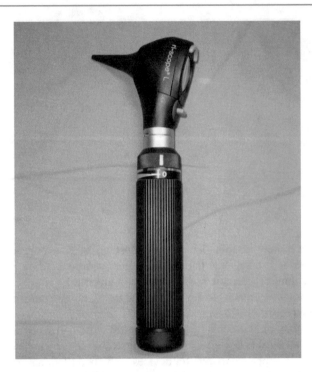

Fig. 1.1 A monocular otoscope gives a two-dimensional view to the EAC and ear drum. It consists of a handle and a head. A light source is integrated in the head. A disposable plastic speculum is attached to the front. A magnifying lens can be used on the rear of the otoscope and gives a triple higher magnification. The lens can also be removed, allowing the experienced examiner to insert an instrument through the otoscope to remove the cerumen. A pneumatic otoscope includes a pump capable of puffing air in order to observe the mobility of the tympanic membrane. Otoscopes can be wall-mounted or portable. Portable models are powered by batteries, which can be rechargeable, the wall-mounted otoscopes are attached to a base that serves as a power source. Alternatively, the otoscope can also be used for examination of a patient's nose and, with the speculum removed, for illuminating the oral cavity

Fig. 1.2 A tele-otoscope is a miniature telescope enabling a good wide-angled overview of the ear drum. It has good illumination and resolution. The diameter of the optics is usually 2.7 mm. A cold light source is needed

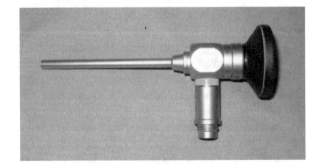

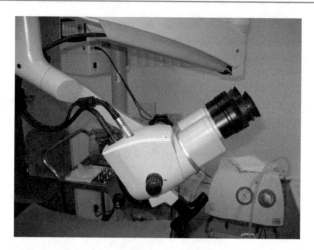

Fig. 1.3 Ambulatory microscope with an integrated camera, used with reusable metal ear specula. The examination is routinely performed by otorhinolaryngologists. The patient is usually supine with the head tilted. The examiner has both hands free and can easily clean and aspirate the contents of the EAC. The binocular view gives the examiner a perception of depth. The picture can be enlarged up to 40 times. In larger magnifications it is also possible to observe the movements of the ear drum such as the in paraganglioma tumours. The supine position also enables the physician to perform smaller procedures. Aspiration to clean the radical cavities can result in vertigo which lasts for a few minutes

Fig. 1.4 Reusable ear specula of different sizes

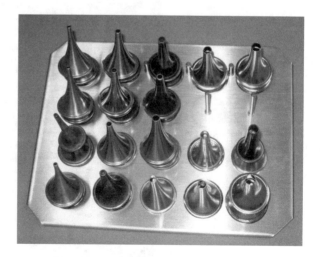

Ear specula with varying diameters (Fig. 1.4) are used to overcome the narrow isthmus of the external ear canal (EAC). We should choose the widest speculum that still allows us to pass the isthmus. The choice of which speculum to pick for the task becomes easier with experience. Picking the right speculum is especially important when examining children. Trying an oversized speculum could injure the delicate skin of the ear canal and should be avoided. If the speculum is too small, it will be very difficult to see the structures in the ear canal or the drum and impossible to clean the ear canal. For cleaning of the EAC we can use curettes of different sizes (for example Buck ear curettes) (Fig. 1.5), forceps for the harder material, and an aspirator for the removal of any secretions (Fig. 1.6).

In the general practitioner's practice, an otoscopy can be restricted by the accumulation of cerumen. Cleaning can be performed by syringing the EAC with water that has been warmed previously to body temperature.

For a correct diagnosis at least 75% of the ear drum should be visible [3], but at least the key structure—the posterior superior quadrant.

Fig. 1.5 Curettes and forceps for cleaning the EAC

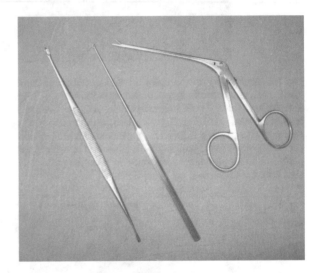

Fig. 1.6 Aspirator extensions of different diameters for suctioning of secretions in the EAC and operative cavities

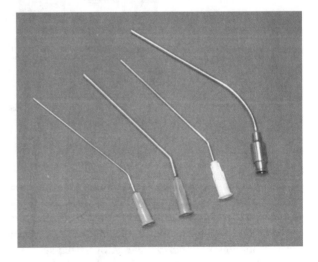

Fig. 1.7 An otoscopic picture displayed on the monitor

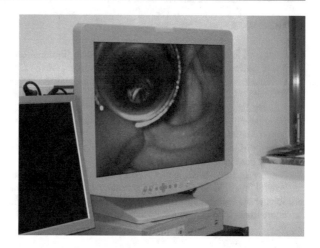

Ideally the otoscopy picture should be documented. This is especially important before and after surgery, when explaining the disease and the therapeutic plan to the patient. In practice a camera integrated into the microscope and connected to a monitor is used. Otoscopic pictures can be stored and also enlarged (Fig. 1.7). Presenting the images on the monitor is also useful for educational purposes.

In children the EAC is much narrower and the child might also be restless. The investigation should be performed as swiftly as possible. Uncertainty in the diagnosis may lead to wrong treatment decisions. In children the overdiagnosis of acute otitis media (AOM) can lead to unnecessary antibiotics prescription, possibly leading to the development of antibiotic resistance, and also carries possible risks of side effects. On the other hand, incorrect or delayed diagnosis when middle ear cholesteatoma or chronic otitis is overlooked may lead to complications such as mastoiditis, meningitis, or other intracranial complications. With conventional otoscopy general practitioners diagnose AOM with 67% accuracy in children younger than 2 years and 75% accuracy in children older than two [4].

It is also possible to attach the camera to the otoscope to depict the EAC and ear drum. Video-otoscopy might provide better interpretation of pathologic ear conditions because of the possibility of consultation. It may also be useful in telemedicine, especially in areas with poor medical coverage [5]. However, a good knowledge of otoscopy is still needed to interpret the findings.

A smartphone otoscopy can be performed by attaching a modified otoscope head (available online) to the camera of an existing smartphone. The technology was developed with the idea of using this method in the paediatric population, where parents could capture images and send them to an otolaryngologist for diagnosis. Studies evaluating the use of smartphone otoscopy have found that only trained healthcare professionals were able to capture useful images, not parents. Nevertheless, such technology might prevent unnecessary emergency or primary care visits [6].

References

1. Barriga F, Schwartz RH, Hayden GF. Adequate illumination for otoscopy. Variations due to power source, bulb, and head and speculum design. Am J Dis Child. 1986;140:1237–40.
2. Pichichero ME. Acute otitis media: Part I. Improving diagnostic accuracy. Am Fam Physician. 2000;61(7):2051–6.
3. Agence Française de Sécurité Sanitaire des Produits de Santé. Antibiotherapie par voie generale en practice courante dans les infections respiratoires hautes de l'adulte et de infant. Argumentaire. 2011:14.
4. Jensen PM, Lous J. Criteria, performance and diagnostic problems in diagnosing acute otitis media. Fam Pract. 1999;16(3):262–8.
5. Damery L, Lescane E, Reffet K, Aussedat C, Bakhos D. Interest of video-otoscopy for the general practicioner. Eur Ann Otorhinolaryngol Head Neck Dis. 2019;136(1):13–7.
6. Schafer A, Hudson S, Elmaraghy CA. Telemedicine in pediatric otolaryngology: ready for prime time? Int J Pediatr Otorhinolaryngol. 2020;138:110399.

Middle Ear Anatomy

The ear is a compound organ sensitive to sound and to the effects of gravity and motion. It consists of the external ear (*auris externa*), the middle ear (*auris media*), and the inner ear (*auris interna*). The inner ear consists of the cochlea, the utriculus, and the sacculus in the vestibule and of three semicircular canals.

The main feature of the middle ear is the tympanic cavity, a small air-containing chamber in the petrous portion of the temporal bone. The middle ear communicates with the nasopharynx through the Eustachian tube and with the mastoid cells through the antrum; that is why the shape and structure of the drum may differ widely depending on the middle ear pressure.

The tympanic membrane (*membrana tympani*) or ear drum serves as a partition between the EAC and tympanic cavity. The membrane is elliptic, measuring 9–10 mm along its major axis and a diameter of 8–9 mm on its minor axis. The membrane varies in form, size, and obliquity. Its external aspect is slightly concave due to the traction of the manubrium of the malleus. The most depressed point is known as the *umbo membranae tympani* and corresponds to the tip of the manubrium. A mallear prominence is formed by the lateral process of the malleus. From there the anterior and posterior malleolar folds (*plica mallearis anterior* and *posterior*) extend to the tympanic sulcus in the anterior and posterior directions. The triangular area bound by the plicae is the flaccid portion (*pars flaccida*) or Shrapnell's membrane. It is attached directly onto the petrous bone [1]. The larger part of the tympanic membrane under the pars flaccida is called the *pars tensa*. It is attached by the fibrocartilaginous ring (*annulus fibrocartilaginous*) to the tympanic sulcus of the temporal bone (Fig. 2.1).

The tympanic membrane is between 50 and 90 μm thick and consists of three layers: the outer (cutaneous) layer, the inner (mucosal) layer, and the fibrous *lamina propria* between them. In the pars flaccida the fibrous layer is absent and it is due to this that, when there is negative pressure in the middle ear, the retraction first develops in the pars flaccida of the ear drum.

The rim of the ear drum is formed by the *annulus tympanicus*, a fibrocartilaginous thickening. It is located in the groove called the *sulcus tympanicus*. In the

J. Rebol, *Otoscopy Findings*, https://doi.org/10.1007/978-3-031-03979-9_2

Fig. 2.1 Right ear. The normal tympanic membrane is translucent, in the level of annulus, with the reflex at the anteroinferior quadrant. *AS* anterosuperior quadrant, *AI* anteroinferior quadrant, *PS* posterosuperior quadrant, *PI* posteroinferior quadrant, *PF* posterior malleolar fold, *LP* lateral process of malleus (mallear prominence), *M* manubrium of malleus, *R* reflex, *A* annulus, *SM* Shrapnell's membrane

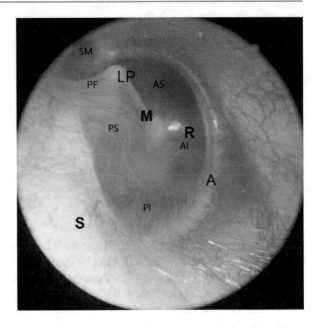

upper part the annulus tympanicus is absent. This is the notch of Rivinus. The outer part of the ear drum is innervated by a branch of the auriculotemporal nerve and the auricular branch of the vagus nerve. The inner part of the ear drum is innervated by the Jacobson's nerve, a branch of the glossopharyngeal nerve.

The arterial supply comes from the deep auricular and anterior tympanic arteries, both of which are branches of the maxillary artery.

In the posterosuperior part of the medial wall of the middle ear, the oval, and the round window niches can be identified (Figs. 2.2 and 2.3).

The bottom of the oval window niche forms the footplate of the *stapes*. The stapes is the smallest ossicle in the body and consists of a base or footplate connected to the head with an anterior and a posterior crus. From the head the stapedial muscle is connected to the pyramidal process (*eminentia pyramidalis*).

The *sinus tympani* is delimited superiorly by the *ponticulus*, running from the pyramidal eminence and promontory. Inferiorly it is limited by *subiculum*. The sinus tympani varies in the posterior extension, but never communicates with the mastoid cells [2]. Even in cases of total perforation of the ear drum, the sinus tympani is difficult to see because it is located beneath the posterior wall of the EAC. The oval window niche can be seen in total and subtotal perforation. Anterior to the oval window is the promontory with the basal turn of the cochlea. Superior to the oval window niche is the horizontal (tympanic) segment of the facial nerve, usually covered with thin bone. Sometimes the facial canal is dehiscent and the nerve bulges over the oval window, a fact important in middle ear surgery because of the possibility of injury.

The round window niche is located anteroinferior to the subiculum and posteroinferior to the promontory. The round window membrane lies in the depth of the

Fig. 2.2 Right ear. Medial wall of the middle ear after removal of the tympanic membrane. *I* incus, *S* head of stapes, *F* tympanic part of the facial nerve (in the bony canal), *PC* cochleariform processus, *M* malleus, *O* oval niche, *R* round window niche, *P* promontory

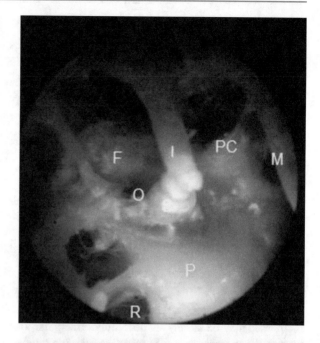

Fig. 2.3 Left ear. Medial wall of the middle ear after removal of the ear drum. *I* incus, *S* head of stapes, *MS* stapedial muscle (musculus stapedius), *Po* ponticulus, *St* sinus tympani, *Su* subiculum, *F* facial nerve, *M* malleus, *O* oval window niche, *R* round window niche, *P* promontory, *H* hypotympanic cells

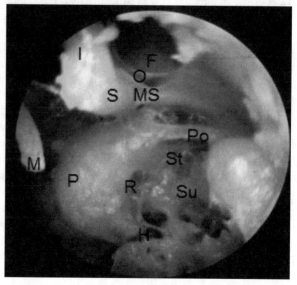

niche. Usually it is oriented horizontally and is frequently obscured by the mucosal veil (Fig. 2.4). The round window membrane can be the site of a perilymphatic fistula (PLF), an abnormal tear or defect in the membrane. It is also the most important structure in cochlear implantation and has to be identified during cochlear implant surgery. It is important to distinguish the round window from the subcochlear canaliculus, which communicates with cells in the petrous apex. Round window

Fig. 2.4 Right ear. Round window niche covered with a thin mucosa. It can be identified in a patient with atelectasis of the ear drum in adhesive otitis media

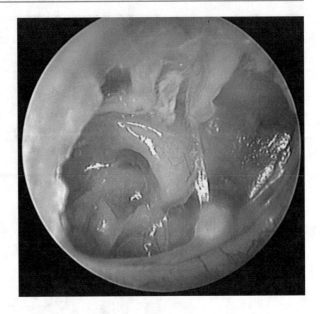

membrane may be kidney shaped, round, triangular, oval, or semilunar. The thickness of the membrane is 60 µm and is, like the tympanic membrane, made up of three layers. The length of the membrane is about 1.7 mm and the width 1.35 mm. The entrance to the round window niche measures 2.2 mm.

Located under the malleus is the *processus cochleariformis*, the origin of the tensor tympani muscle, which is attached to the manubrium of malleus. The hypotympanic cells are situated under the promontory.

The *tympanic ostium* of the Eustachian tube is located in the anterior wall of the tympanic cavity, a few millimetres above the floor (Fig. 2.5). The Eustachian tube ventilates, clears, and protects the tympanic cavity. The fibrocartilaginous portion makes up two thirds of the 35 mm long tube. The bony part lies lateral to the internal carotid artery.

The tympanic cavity is traversed by the *chorda tympani*, which carries gustatory fibres for the anterior two thirds of the tongue. It arises from the facial nerve. The course of the facial nerve in the temporal bone is divided into four segments, the labyrinthine part being the shortest. It is only 4 mm long and extends from the entrance in the fallopian canal to the geniculate ganglion. The horizontal (tympanic) part of the facial nerve directly overlies the oval window niche and the cochleariform process and is 13 mm long (Fig. 2.6). At the sinus tympani, the nerve turns into the mastoid segment, forming the second genu.

The ossicular chain transmits sound from the ear drum to the cochlea. The malleus weights 25 mg, the incus 27 mg, and the stapes 3 mg. The malleus is the lateralmost ossicle and is incorporated in the ear drum (Fig. 2.7). It consists of the head, the manubrium, and the lateral process. The body of the incus and head of the malleus articulate in the attic (*epitympanum*). The long process of the incus stretches inferiorly, paralleling the manubrium, and terminates in the lenticular

Fig. 2.5 Right ear. Normal transparent ear drum. The incudostapedial joint with the stapedial muscle can be identified under the posterosuperior quadrant of the ear drum

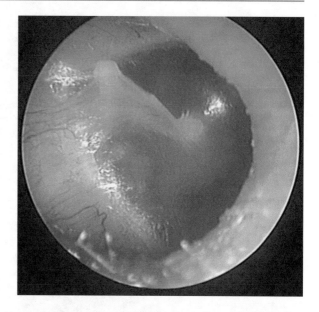

Fig. 2.6 Right ear. Tympanic orifice of the Eustachian tube under the intact ear drum (arrow)

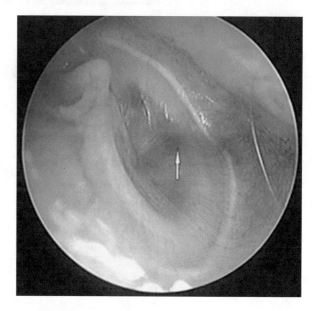

process, which articulates with the stapes (Figs. 2.8 and 2.9). The long process of the incus is the first part of the ossicles that is resorbed in chronic otitis due to its tenuous blood supply. The stapes consists of two crura, the head and the footplate, which seals the oval window (Fig. 2.10). The stapedial muscle stretches from the pyramidal process to the superior aspect of the posterior crus and the head of the stapes.

Fig. 2.7 Left ear.
Dehiscent horizontal part
of the facial nerve (black
arrow). The patient had
been operated in the past
for cholesteatoma of the
middle ear, which
destroyed the bone
overlying the facial nerve

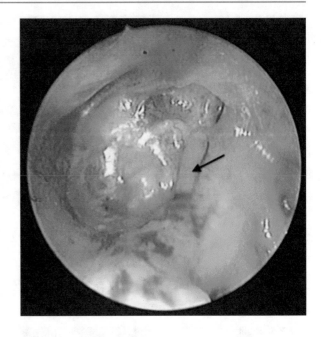

Fig. 2.8 The right malleus

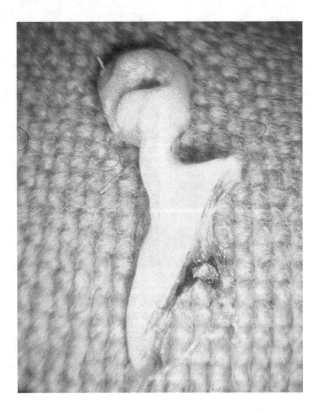

Fig. 2.9 The right incus: *L* processus lenticularis, *PL* processus longus (long process), *C* corpus, *PB* processus breve (short process)

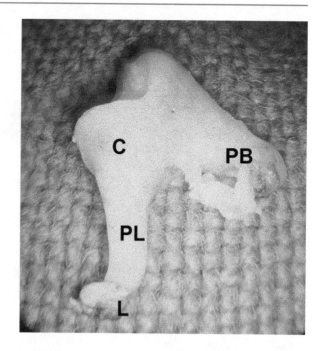

Fig. 2.10 Suprastructure of the stapes removed at stapedotomy, placed for size comparison on a 1 euro cent coin, which has a diameter of 16 mm. The anterior and posterior crura as well as the head of stapes can be identified in the suprastructure. The stapes measures 3 × 2.5 mm

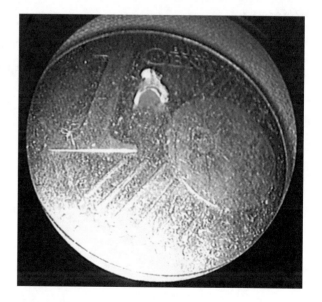

Sometimes we may also observe a high riding jugular bulb, where a roof of the jugular bulb extends more superiorly in the temporal bone as normal, and may appear as a blue lesion behind the intact ear drum (Fig. 2.11).

Fig. 2.11 High jugular bulbus. The ear drum has a dark red appearance in the inferior quadrants. The jugular bulb might be dehiscent without bone covering (sigmoid plate) and any myringotomy in this case would result in heavy bleeding. The condition can easily be recognised on contrast-enhanced CT

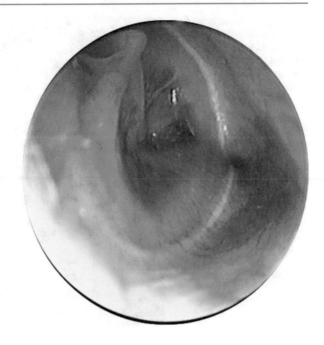

References

1. Anson BJ, Donaldson JA. Surgical anatomy of the temporal bone and ear. 2nd ed. Philadelphia: W. B. Saunders; 1973. p. 153–73.
2. Gulya AJ. Anatomy and embryology of the ear. In: Hughes GB, Pensak ML, editors. Clinical otology. 3rd ed. New York: Thieme; 2007. p. 3–34.

Diseases of the External Auditory Canal

3

The external ear consists of the auricle and the external ear canal (*meatus acusticus externus*). The medial boundary of the external ear is the tympanic membrane. In adults the length of the EAC is approximately 2.5 cm. The lateral third of the EAC consists of cartilage that is angled downward and forward in relation to the bony inner two thirds of the EAC. The entrance in the EAC is called *porus acusticus externus*.

During otoscopy the mobile cartilaginous part has to be pulled upward and backward in order for us to see the eardrum and the medial part of the EAC. The medial part of the EAC is formed by the tympanic part of the temporal bone. The skin in the medial part of the EAC directly covers the periosteum without subcutaneous tissue. The medial part is much more vulnerable to the injuries, which can also occur during cleaning or even during the insertion of the ear speculum during the otoscopy.

Located in front of the cartilaginous part of the EAC is the parotid gland. Infections such as external necrotizing otitis might spread towards the parotid gland. Anterior to the bony part of the EAC is the temporomandibular joint. After fracture of the anterior part of the EAC, a scab and blood can be seen in the EAC. Posterior to the EAC is the mastoid consisting of mastoid cells. The degree of pneumatisation of the mastoid varies and is influenced by previous inflammations. In mastoiditis the skin of the posterior EAC is swollen.

Desquamated skin migrates from the medial part of the EAC towards meatus. Secretions of ceruminal glands moisten the EAC, repel water and are bacteriostatic.

3.1 Cerumen

Cerumen (Figs. 3.1, 3.2, and 3.3) is a product of the ceruminal glands, which are located in the outer two thirds of the EAC. It has an acidic pH and protects the skin against inflammation. Tiny hairs inside the EAC propagate cerumen towards the meatus. Sometimes this function fails and cerumen accumulates in the EAC, which

© The Author(s), under exclusive license to Springer Nature
Switzerland AG 2022
J. Rebol, *Otoscopy Findings*, https://doi.org/10.1007/978-3-031-03979-9_3

Fig. 3.1 Left ear. Ceruminal scales predominately on the posterior wall in the outer part of the EAC. In the medial part, the scale covers the eardrum

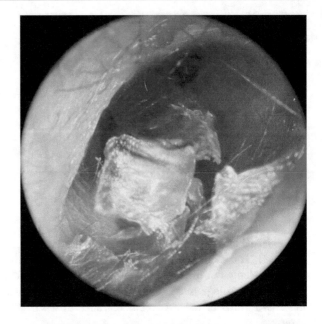

Fig. 3.2 Left ear. The entire lumen of the EAC is filled with cerumen. The eardrum cannot be seen

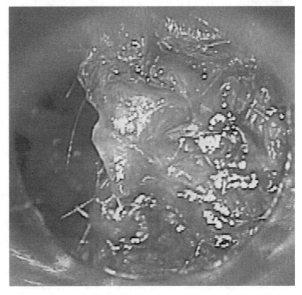

then needs to be cleaned. Patients often use cotton buds to remove cerumen, but by doing so tend to merely propagate the cerumen further into the EAC. Especially in children this makes the cleaning of the EAC more difficult.

Cerumen has different appearance in different races.

Fig. 3.3 Left ear. Stenotic EAC with cerumen. Patiens with stenosis in the middle part of the EAC often get a buildup of cerumen. Removal of such cerumen can be difficult and specialist instruments are usually needed

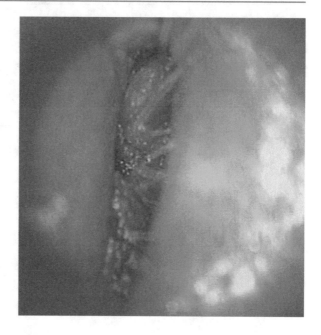

Cerumen can be cleaned manually with instruments under the microscope (in the ENT practice), it can be aspirated or syringed with water at body temperature. If the water used for syringing is to cold or to warm, the patient may feel dizzy (like performing the caloric test).

Important note: contraindications for syringing are eardrum perforation, chronic ear inflammation, and conditions after ear operations such as modified radical mastoidectomy or radical mastoidectomy.

3.2 Cysts of the EAC

Cysts appear mostly in the lateral part of the EAC (Fig. 3.4). In the procedure of differential diagnosis, we have to consider an atheroma, perichondritis, benign or malignant tumours. A biopsy is advisable for such conditions.

Epidermoid cysts are benign findings caused by inflammation of hair cortex follicles and proliferation of epidermal cells within the dermis or superficial subcutaneous tissue [1]. Such cysts are filled with keratin and lined with stratified squamous epithelium.

Destruction of the bone by an epidermal cyst does not occur often. Although it has been suggested that epidermoid cyst and cholesteatoma are the same disease, they behave in slightly different ways. They are indistinguishable histopathologically and radiologically. Usually they grow slowly and may complicate as abscesses, with haemorrhage and malignant transformation.

Fig. 3.4 Left ear. A cyst at the entrance of the EAC, completely obstructing the lumen

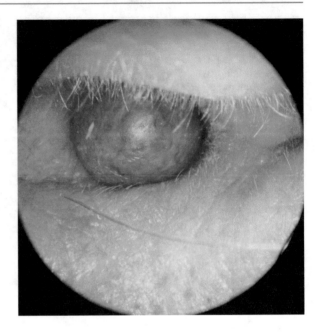

3.3   Exostoses and Osteoma

Exostoses are bony accumulations in the bony part of the EAC located in the inner third of the EAC (Figs. 3.5, 3.6, 3.7, and 3.8). They are often multiple and bilateral. They can vary in size and shape—they can be round or elongated. They are caused by chronic irritation, which can be physical, chemical, or thermal [2]. Most frequently they are found in divers and swimmers with exposition to cold sea water for at least 10 years. The cause of the new bone formation is probably prolonged vasodilatation that follows cold water exposure. The condition is more common in coastal regions and is known as the "surfer's ear" and has a male predominance.

Exostoses can arise in the area from the tympanic ring to the isthmus of the EAC. When the exostoses are small, they are asymptomatic, but once they grow to a certain size, they may significantly reduce the lumen of the EAC and cause external otitis. They might also cause conductive hearing loss because of cerumen impaction in the narrow EAC. In some cases, they can completely obstruct the EAC also causing conductive hearing loss. Patients often have otitis externa, especially if they are exposed to water. In such cases, an operation may be indicated. In the procedure the skin is preserved and moved medially. The bone is drilled away and the skin is put back in its original position. It is important to preserve all the skin, because this way postoperative healing is faster.

Osteoma is a benign neoplasm of the bony EAC (Figs. 3.9, 3.10, and 3.11). It is often pedunculated and is found unilaterally. An osteoma usually arises in the vicinity of the petrotympanic or tympanomastoid fissure lateral to the isthmus and does not have a history of chronic irritation. It can be distinguished from exostoses histologically.

Fig. 3.5 Left ear. Round exostoses on the posterior and anterior wall. They are already touching in the inferior part of the EAC. Only a small part of the eardrum can be seen (posterosuperior quadrant with handle of malleus). The patient had a history of several external otitides and chose to have an operation

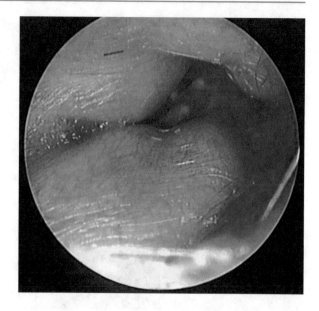

Fig. 3.6 Left ear. Narrow EAC due to elongated exostoses in the anterior and posterior wall. A small round exostosis has also appeared on the superior wall. The eardrum cannot be seen. During water exposure, water can reach the area of the EAC beyond the stenosis, but has difficulty escaping through the stenosis

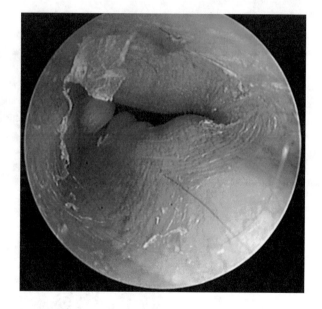

Fig. 3.7 Right ear.
Extensive exostoses which
completely obstructed the
EAC. The patient had
problems with repeated
infections of the EAC and
also had conductive
hearing loss in the latter
months. A complete
obstruction of the EAC is
more difficult to operate
because of the preservation
of the skin of the EAC

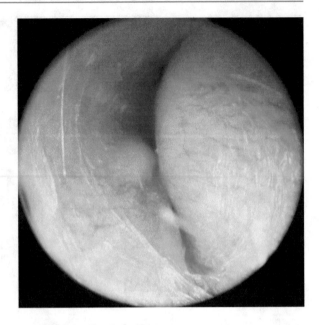

Fig. 3.8 Right ear.
Extensive exostoses, which
almost completely obstruct
the EAC. There is still
some lumen superiorly

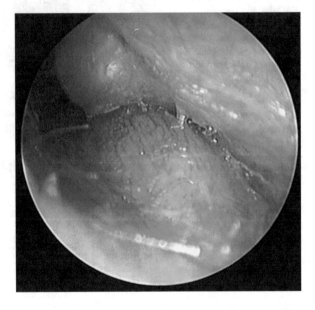

Fig. 3.9 Right ear. EAC osteoma, which is totally obstructing the lumen. The patient's hearing deteriorated, when the EAC was completely occluded. Osteoma can be removed with a small chisel under local anaesthesia, disconnecting it from its base

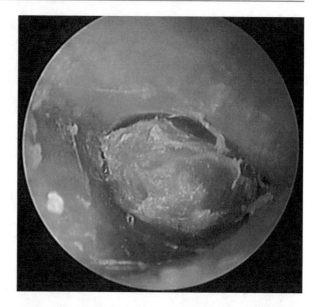

Fig. 3.10 Left ear. A smaller osteoma on the posterior wall of the EAC. Removal is even easier under local anaesthesia, because it is not difficult to identify its base

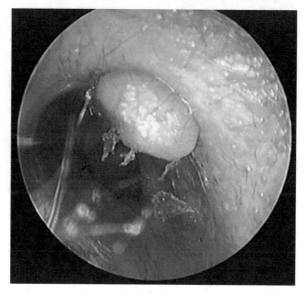

3.4 Foreign Bodies in the External Ear Canal

Foreign bodies can enter EAC in various ways. Children, either themselves or their peers, can put parts of plastic toys in the EAC. Foreign bodies can also come from the nature (e.g. pussy willow catkins).

Foreign bodies may enter the EAC in work-related incidents. Metal foreign bodies (Figs. 3.12 and 3.13) or tree branches may injure the EAC skin or even perforate the eardrum.

Fig. 3.11 Left ear. Osteoma in the posterior part of the middle ear. Osteoma might obstruct the access to the oval window niche during stapes surgery. It is also possible that it limits the mobility of the ossicular chain, causing the conductive hearing loss

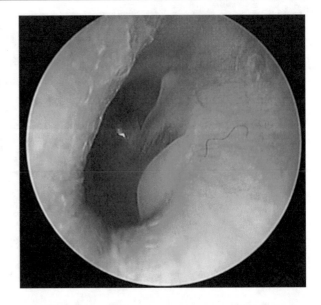

Fig. 3.12 Left ear. Aluminium alloy entered the EAC during a production process. At the examination, the patient had a strong pain due to burns to the skin and eardrum

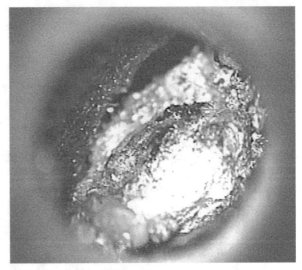

If the foreign body is small and we can see that the eardrum is intact (Figs. 3.14, 3.15, and 3.16), we can syringe the EAC. With larger foreign bodies (Figs. 3.17, 3.18, 3.19, and 3.20), removal with a hook or curette is usually necessary. This should be advanced medially of the foreign body and then pulled out of the EAC together with the foreign body. Care has to be taken not to injure the eardrum. After removal of the foreign body, the eardrum should be inspected for perforation.

In adults the most common foreign body is cotton wool, which can be left behind in the EAC, often by the patients during attempts to clean the EAC. In cases of

Fig. 3.13 Left ear. The same patient as in Fig. 3.19 after the removal of the aluminium alloy from the EAC. The skin of the EAC is swollen, there is a total perforation of the eardrum. The patient also had partial facial nerve paralysis

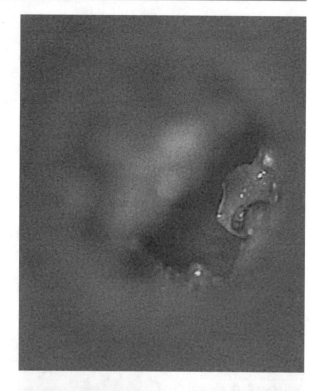

Fig. 3.14 Right ear. Initial exostoses on the anterior and posterior walls of the EAC. Hair, which is touching the eardrum and in doing so causing discomfort to the patient, can be observed in the EAC

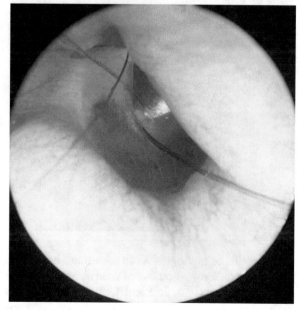

Fig. 3.15 Right ear.
Plastic pellet in the medial
part of the EAC in front of
the eardrum. The foreign
body was discovered
accidentally

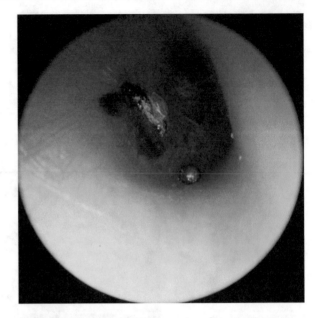

Fig. 3.16 Left ear. Small
metal pieces which entered
the EAC during welding on
the anterior and inferior
wall of the EAC. A small
round exostosis can also be
seen on the ceiling

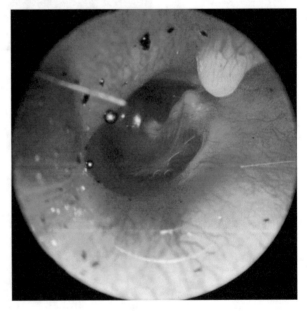

chronic otitis or myringitis it can sometimes become soaked with pus. The second
most common foreign bodies that need removal from the EAC are parts of ear plugs.

Living insects (Figs. 3.21 and 3.22) can also enter the EAC. They move towards
the eardrum and the strokes of their wings and other movement are very unpleasant
for the patient.

Fig. 3.17 Left ear. Parts
of silicone ear protection.
The patient used silicone
ear protection to go
swimming but was unable
to remove the silicone
afterwards. Some patients
with chronic ear conditions
and after operations are
instructed to protect their
ear from water. Earplugs
can also be custom made

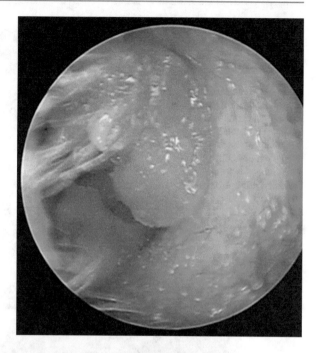

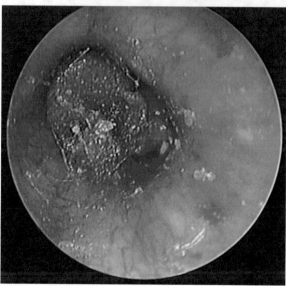

Fig. 3.18 Left ear. A blue piece of silicone in the medial part of the EAC. Silicone may be applied
to the EAC to make a cast as a base for the model for a hearing aid. If the EAC is narrow, silicone
can sometimes remain in the medial part of the EAC

Fig. 3.19 Right ear. While playing, the child put a plastic pellet in the EAC. During an attempt to remove the foreign body by the primary care physician, the EAC was injured. The EAC skin is swollen and is bleeding, which makes the removal even more difficult. The foreign body is located medially, just in front of the eardrum

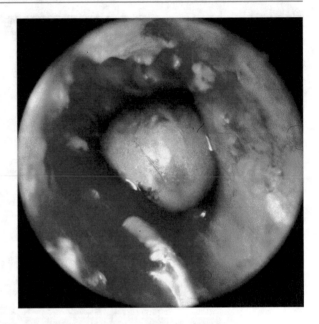

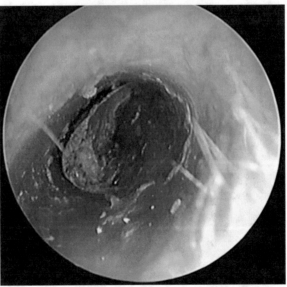

Fig. 3.20 Left ear. Visible in the medial part of the EAC is a piece of concrete. The concrete was strongly adherent to the eardrum. The patient was a construction worker, who was exposed to a burst of fluid concrete entering his EAC. When the mass hardened, it was possible to remove most of it from the EAC but some remained on the eardrum. After instillation of topical anaesthetic (lidocaine spray), the remainder of the foreign body was removed preserving the integrity of the eardrum. The patient was advised to prevent water entering the EAC for 2 weeks and was able to return to work the same day

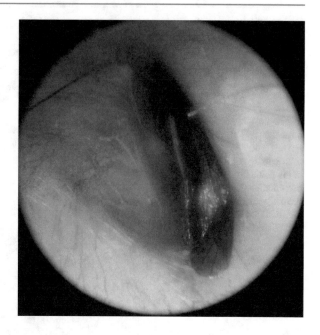

Fig. 3.21 Right ear. A moth in the medial part of the EAC. The patient was watching a football game when the insect entered the ear canal. At home he poured water into the EAC and the unpleasant sensations disappeared, probably when the moth died and stopped moving

Complications after foreign body removal include: laceration of the external auditory canal, tympanic membrane perforation, external otitis, and hematomas [3].

In a study by Tiago et al. 40% of foreign bodies were removed with alligator forceps, 32% with irrigation, 14% with a curette, and in 14% more than one method was needed [4].

Success in removing an EAC foreign body depends on size, shape, and texture of the foreign body, the cooperation of the patient at time of removal, the ability to visualise the foreign body and surrounding structures, and any trauma to the ear from insertion or attempted removals. Equipment as well as the experience and skill of the individual attempting the removal are also important [5]. Indications for referral to otomicroscopy are spherical or sharp-edged objects, disk batteries, and vegetable matter foreign body, location adjacent to tympanic membrane, foreign body in the ear for more than 24 h, child younger than four, difficulty in visualisation and previous removal attempts. Otomicroscopic guided attempts have higher success rate, especially in patients younger than four. Beside better visibility with the microscope, the variety of instruments also plays an important role in removal of foreign bodies from the EAC.

3.5 Bullous Myringitis

Bullous myringitis is a common condition characterised by vesicles or bullae on the eardrum without affecting the middle ear (Figs. 3.23, 3.24, 3.25, and 3.26). A sudden haemorrhagic discharge occurs when a bulla ruptures spontaneously, this is also followed by an easing of pain. Bullous myringitis is thought to be caused by viruses

Fig. 3.22 Left ear. Housefly larvae known as maggots. The eggs resemble grains of rice and after a day hatch into larvae. They are legless and feed from the egg-laying site for 3–5 days. The patient was a farmer, who accidentally got a housefly in his EAC. During presentation the larvae were alive and moved constantly in the medial part of the EAC

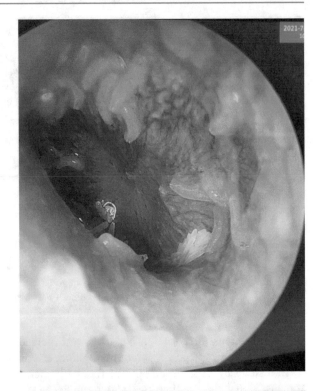

Fig. 3.23 Right ear. The eardrum is swollen in the posterior part, a bulla is located in the central portion of the eardrum. The bulla if filled with serous fluid

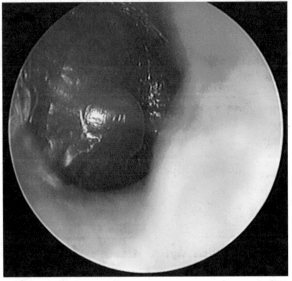

(respiratory syncytial virus or influenza) although *Streptococcus pneumoniae* is the most commonly found bacteria [5]. It can also be triggered by *Mycoplasma pneumonia*. The peak incidence of the disease is in winter months and it can be also combined

Fig. 3.24 Left ear. The entire eardrum is covered with a haemorrhagic bulla, which has not perforated yet. The patient had otalgia and upper respiratory tract infection

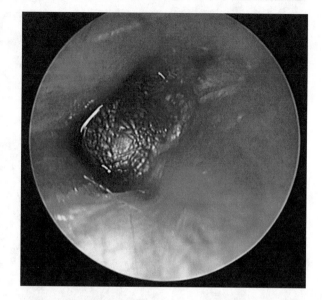

Fig. 3.25 Right ear. Larger confluent haemorrhagic bullae on the posterior part of the eardrum. Spontaneous rupture resulting in haemorrhagic otorrhea can occur

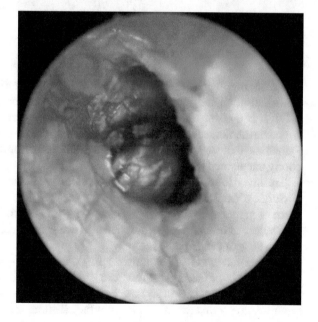

with acute otitis media (AOM). The disease is often accompanied by fever and otalgia. Patients may have conductive hearing loss in presence of effusion and sensorineural loss is also possible. Pure tone audiometry is therefore necessary in these patients. Sensorineural hearing loss completely recovers in approximately 60% of patients [6, 7].

High doses of amoxicillin or macrolide antibiotics (for mycoplasma infection) are recommended as well as analgesics. The disease usually heals without any sequelae.

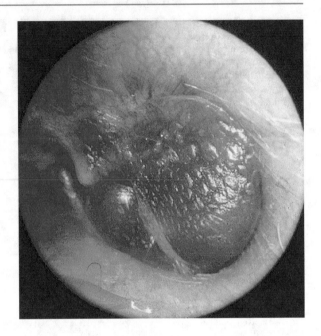

3.6   Granular Myringitis

Granular myringitis is a chronic disorder characterised by squamous de-epithelialisation and granulation of the tympanic membrane (Figs. 3.27, 3.28, and 3.29). It is a result of localised chronic inflammation of the lateral surface of the tympanic membrane. Lesions can also be seen on the EAC skin close to the annulus. Symptoms include chronic otorrhea and mild discomfort in the ear. The disease is poorly understood [8].

Treatment is exclusively local. Patients also have to avoid water entering the EAC.

Surgical excision of granulation tissue resulted in an 80% reduction of recurrence of granular myringitis when compared with conventional antibiotic therapy. Topical use of diluted vinegar solution also achieved a reduction of granular myringitis in 96% of cases.

In some patients the condition may progress towards stenosis or even postinflammatory atresia of the EAC (Figs. 3.30, 3.31, 3.32, 3.33, and 3.34). In such cases surgical therapy (canaloplasty) can be performed. The stenotic and atretic tissue is removed, preserving the middle layer of the eardrum, and the defect is covered with a skin graft. Long-term results are still not always satisfactory and restenosis can occur.

In histologic sections of the resected ear canal skin from the osseous part of the EAC it was found that the ectopic apocrine glands with accumulation of the secretions (cerumen) were present. The absence of myoepithelial cells around the acini of the ectopic apocrine glands results in accumulation of cerumen, triggering inflammation of the EAC skin. Better postoperative results can be expected if the

Fig. 3.27 Right ear. Initial phase of chronic granulomatous myringitis. There is a defect in the epithelial lining in the anterior part of the eardrum. Granulation tissue can begin to grow in this area

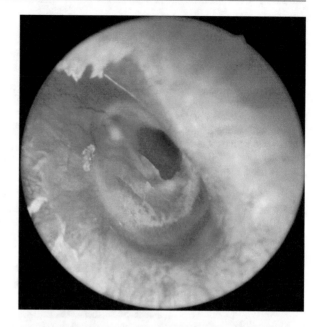

Fig. 3.28 Right ear. Another example of chronic myringitis with the defect in the anteroinferior quadrant of the eardrum. The defect also extends to the ear canal skin. Dried secretions can be seen on the anterior wall of the EAC

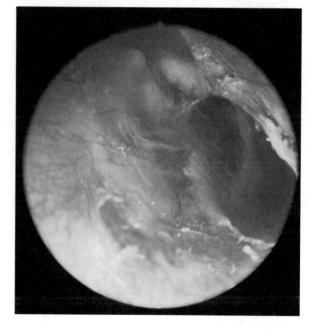

Fig. 3.29 Right ear.
Typical otoscopic finding
in a patient with chronic
myringitis. Granulation
tissue can be seen on the
posterior wall in front of
the eardrum. The eardrum
and especially anterior and
inferior walls of the EAC
are covered with purulent
secretion

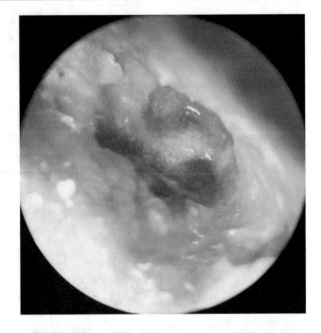

Fig. 3.30 Left ear. The
eardrum is red and
swollen. Almost the whole
eardrum is covered with
granulations. There are
transparent secretions on
the surface, which can
become suppurative

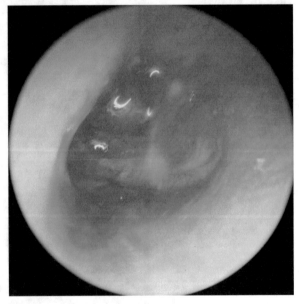

Fig. 3.31 Right ear. The lumen of the EAC is very narrow and the eardrum is no longer visible. Stenosis is one of the sequelae of the growth of granulation tissue, which is very vulnerable and bleeds after cleaning the EAC with aspiration

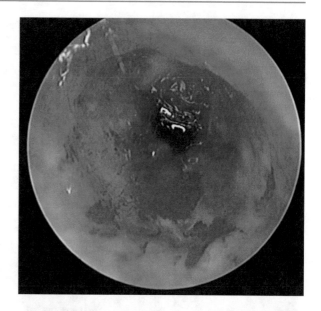

Fig. 3.32 Left ear. Postinflammatory stenosis of the EAC, which is practically impassable due to granulation and fibrosis in the medial part of the EAC

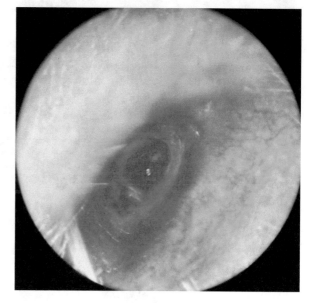

Fig. 3.33 Left ear. False fundus. Due to chronic myringitis the eardrum became thicker and eventually postinflammatory atresia developed. Patients with this condition have conductive hearing loss. Surgical therapy with meticulous excision of diseased pathologic tissue and a subsequent skin graft can be successful

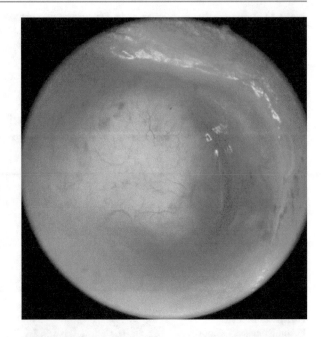

Fig. 3.34 Left ear. Another example of postinflammatory atresia of the EAC with false fundus

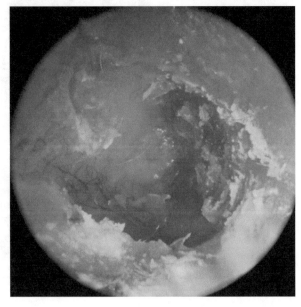

split-thickness skin graft used for the reconstruction does not exceed the thickness of 0.4 mm, which is not containing the apocrine glands. The glands can cause the recurrent stenosis of the EAC [9].

3.7   Osteoradionecrosis

Radiotherapy is used as a primary or adjunctive treatment for many malignancies in the head and neck. Among them tumours of the parotid glands are most common, followed by nasopharyngeal, oral cavity, and skin tumours.

Symptoms can appear after many years. In experiments osteoradionecrosis was noticed as soon as 12 weeks after the initiation of radiotherapy. The average radiation dose in humans which developed osteoradionecrosis was 60 Gy. It seems that there is some causality between higher doses and development of osteoradionecrosis [10]. Patients with osteoradionecrosis would complain about otorrhea, otalgia, hearing loss, which may be conductive or sensorineural. Radiation to the middle ear causes mucosal hypertrophy, loss of ciliary function, ossicular necrosis, and Eustachian tube obstruction. Negative pressure in the middle ear in turn causes secretory otitis media, eardrum atelectasis, cholesteatoma, and chronic inflammation.

Damage to the inner ear may lead to complete hearing loss and patients may become candidates for cochlear implantation.

All patients have exposed necrotic bone and may have fistulae towards the temporomandibular joint and mastoid. Other findings include debris in the EAC, tympanic membrane perforation, cholesteatoma, purulence, otitis externa, granulation tissue, canal stenosis, and middle ear effusion (Figs. 3.35, 3.36, 3.37, 3.38, and 3.39).

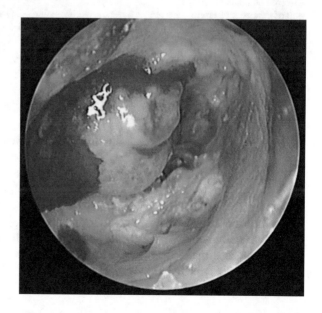

Fig. 3.35 Left ear. The patient had a malignant tumour of the parotid gland (*mucoepidermoid carcinoma*). She was operated (total parotidectomy) and subsequently received radiotherapy. She has severe problems with trismus because of the changes in her temporomandibular joint. At first presentation a large granulation tissue was found in front of the eardrum, the EAC was covered with suppurative discharge

Fig. 3.36 Left ear. The same patient as in the previous figure. After removal of the granulation tissue and local therapy, the discharge was not as evident, but granulation tissue is still present in the front part of the ear. Major surgery in these patients has to be avoided because of vascularisation problems. Healing is impaired because of poor vascularisation after the radiotherapy

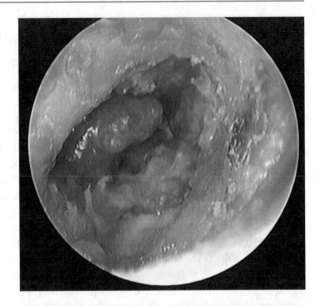

Fig. 3.37 Left ear. The same patient as in the previous figures. The final stage after the local therapy. The ear is dry, there is no granulation tissue in front of the eardrum. Dehiscence with necrotic bone can be observed on the posterior wall of the EAC. Necrotic bone is removed from time to time during aural toileting

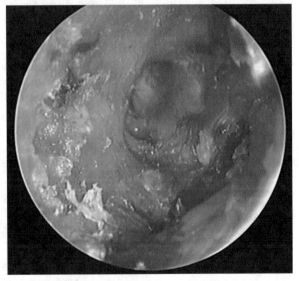

The overall agreement is that therapy should be conservative in local osteoradionecrosis. Potential benefits in terms of symptom relief should be carefully weighed against the risks of surgery within the radiated temporal bone.

Cochlear implantation in patients with osteoradionecrosis of the temporal bone is controversial. Irradiated patients often have profound hearing loss or deafness due to intracochlear damage. On the other hand, placing the device in the necrotic field may predispose infectious complications as well as wound healing disorders. Auditory brainstem response audiometry in patients treated with radiotherapy for

Fig. 3.38 Right ear. The patient received radiotherapy because of a malignant nasopharyngeal carcinoma. Patients can have problems with the discharge from the EAC even years after therapy. On the bottom of the picture necrotic bone is exposed on the posterior wall of the EAC

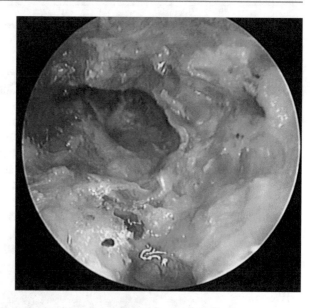

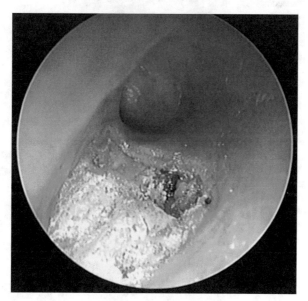

Fig. 3.39 Left ear. Patient after the treatment of nasopharyngeal carcinoma. On the inferior wall of the EAC a large defect with the necrotic bone can be seen. When presented, the patient was completely deaf on both sides. The classical approach through the mastoidectomy and posterior tympanotomy was not possible because of the communication between the EAC and mastoid cells. The necrotic bone was removed, subtotal petrosectomy was performed, and the defect was closed with abdominal fat, after the electrode was inserted into the cochlea. The patient has been followed for many years and their soft tissues and bone are without inflammation

nasopharyngeal carcinoma demonstrated an absence of retrocochlear effects, so they can be candidates for cochlear implantation.

3.8   Herpes Zoster Oticus (Ramsey Hunt Syndrome)

Herpes zoster oticus or Ramsey Hunt syndrome is caused by reactivation of varicella zoster virus in the geniculate ganglion and is characterised by intense otalgia, haemorrhagic vesicles in the eardrum, ear canal, and helix (Figs. 3.40 and 3.41). The vesicles are very painful. Facial nerve paresis can often be observed, also

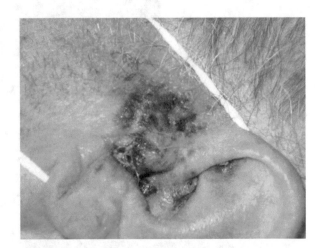

Fig. 3.40 Left ear. Haemorrhagic vesicles in the preauricular region, on the tragus and in the meatus of the EAC. Ramsey Hunt syndrome in immunocompromised patient with leukaemia. The patient had combined hearing loss, vestibular and facial nerve functions were normal

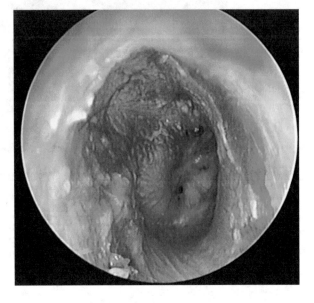

Fig. 3.41 Right ear. Ear canal skin is swollen, eardrum is covered with haemorrhagic vesicles. The patient had herpes zoster oticus with almost total facial nerve paresis

accompanied with sensorineural hearing loss and vertigo. Herpes zoster accounts for about 12% of peripheral facial nerve paresis, which is usually unilateral. Complete recovery of the facial nerve occurs only in 20% of patients. Facial paresis and vesicles do not always appear simultaneously and some patients have paresis several days before the onset of zoster. The virus can also cause facial paresis without skin lesions (zoster sine herpete) and a diagnosis is set by serological investigations [11].

Patients are treated with antiviral drugs, corticosteroids and analgesics [12]. Early onset of therapy within 3 days of the onset of facial palsy is critical. The chances of achieving grade I HB (House Brackman), if the therapy is started 7 days after onset are less than 30%. Early therapy reduces the development of complications, so the early diagnosis is important [13].

3.9   Otomycosis (Mycotic External Otitis)

Otomycosis is more common in warmer months and in tropical regions. Most infections are caused by the *Aspergillus* (*niger* and *fumigatus*) and *Candida albicans* fungi. Unlike Aspergillus infections, Candida infections do not have a characteristic appearance. They can appear as otorrhea that does not respond to local antibiotic therapy. Infection is more common in diabetics and immunocompromised patients with chronical ear discharge. It may also appear in patients who use antibiotic local drops for a longer period. Fungi are opportunists and grow when the bacteria are supressed by antibiotics. Because of that, use of local antibiotics should be limited to 7 days and long-term use avoided.

Patients complain of itching and otalgia as well as conductive hearing loss, when the EAC is filled with mycotic masses (Figs. 3.42, 3.43, 3.44, 3.45, 3.46, and 3.47).

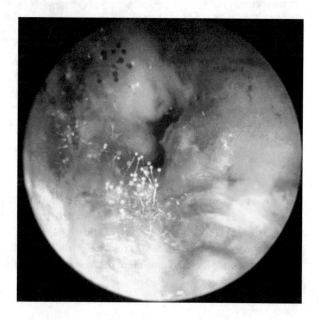

Fig. 3.42 Right ear. The ear canal walls are covered with pus and grey mycotic masses. This is most probably an *Aspergillus niger* infection

Fig. 3.43 Right ear. Mycotic external otitis. The whole EAC is filled with pus with mycotic masses on the anterior canal wall

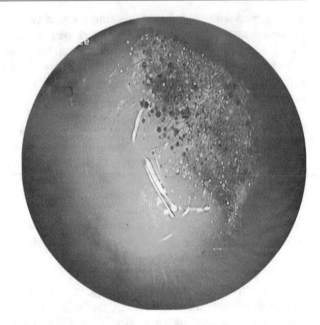

Fig. 3.44 Left ear. Another example of Aspergillus infection. The whole medial part if the EAC and the eardrum are covered with dark mycotic masses. From the appearance we may conclude that we are dealing with an *Aspergillus niger* infection. A drop of pus can also be seen in the middle. Therapy is local with the aspiration of the mycotic masses and application of local antimycotics like clotrimazole or ketoconazole

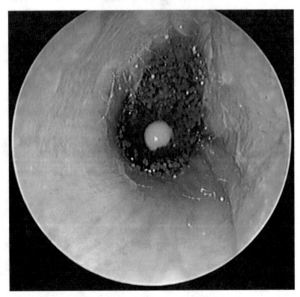

Topical clotrimazole is effective against *Aspergillus* as well as *Candida albicans*. Regular cleaning of the infested EAC is also important. Other therapy options include topical ketoconazole, cresylate otic drops, aluminium acetate otic drops [14].

Otomycosis may be observed relatively often in canal wall down mastoidectomies. Application of local antibiotic drops may change the local environment in the

Fig. 3.45 Right ear. Otomycosis in the medial part of the EAC. The skin of the EAC is swollen and in the medial part the yellowish masses can be seen also covering the eardrum. Beside *Aspergillus* spp., the more frequent causative organism might also be *Candida albicans*

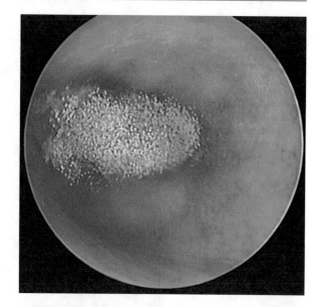

Fig. 3.46 Right ear. Condition after modified radical mastoidectomy. Medially a perforation in the eardrum is visible. The ear is chronically inflamed and the cavity is filled with pus, white masses and some dark conidial heads of Aspergillus. The mycotic infection is most probably a superinfection. The patient had been treated with antibiotic drops, which favour fungal growth. Treatment is local with aspiration and application of antimycotic drops or antiseptic powders

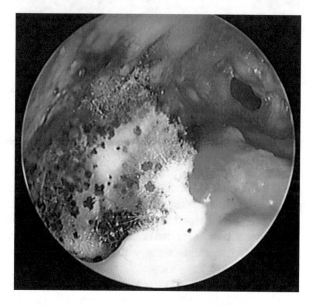

EAC and facilitate nosocomial fungal superinfections. Cerumen production is also altered and the relative humidity in the EAC increased, which favours fungal growth. Eradication of disease is therefore more difficult in the mastoid cavity. Therapy with oral antimycotics is reserved for severe disease that does not response to topical therapy.

Fig. 3.47 Left ear. At larger magnification the conidiophores of Aspergillus can be seen. Colonies of the fungus reproduce from conidiophores and release conidia which are air born. Inhalational exposition of conidia in the environment is continuous. In healthy individuals, conidia are eliminated by respiratory mucosa. Everybody inhales several hundred spores per day

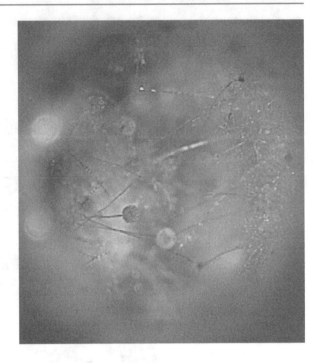

3.10   External Otitis

Patients with EAC eczema or patients with a narrow EAC often have the external otitis. Beside this mechanical trauma, wet environment (swimming in pools) or use of hearing aids also increase the risk of external otitis. It is more common in summer months.

We can distinguish four types of external otitis: acute diffuse external otitis, acute localised (Otitis externa circumscripta), chronic external otitis and necrotizing (malignant) otitis externa. The latter is better indicated as osteomyelitis of the tympanic bone (in the worst case with expansion in the entire temporal bone).

A typical sign of external otitis is pain when pressing on the tragus and during chewing. In fungal infections, we can observe a white or grey layer in the EAC. If the initial therapy fails, a smear might be advisable.

In acute external otitis the most common bacteria is *Pseudomonas aeruginosa* (in about 60%), followed by *Staphylococcus aureus* (in about 20%), *Proteus mirabilis*, *Escherichia coli*, and fungi.

Cleaning of EAC, which can be done with a 3% H_2O_2 solution and daily changing of strips with antibiotics (ciprofloxacin) and corticosteroid ointment is important. External otitis is characterised by oedema of the EAC skin, sometimes the lumen is completely obstructed (Fig. 3.48). Antibiotic solutions with steroids can be applied when the oedema of the EAC resolves (Fig. 3.49). If the EAC is infested with fungi, an antimycotic solution (clotrimazole) should be applied. The therapy for common external otitis is local, systemic antibiotic therapy is not necessary. In case of an involvement of bony structures (see above) an adequate antibiotic regime is mandatory; in some cases an additional surgery is indicated.

Acute local otitis externa represents the inflammation of the hair follicles in the EAC and is known also as furuncle (Fig. 3.50). The pathogen is *Staphylococcus aureus*.

Fig. 3.48 Left ear. The EAC is swollen, very painful, the anterior and posterior EAC walls are touching each other. A strip with antibiotic and corticosteroid cream reduces the oedema of the skin and then antibiotic drops with corticosteroid can be applied

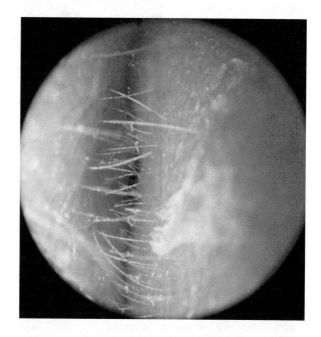

Fig. 3.49 Left ear. The EAC skin is diffusely swollen with a suppurative secretion inside the EAC. The patient had been on holiday at the seaside for several days. Bacteria were isolated in the smear. The patient responded well to the local antibiotic therapy

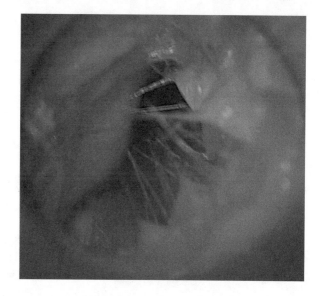

Fig. 3.50 Right ear. Furuncle on the posterior wall at the entrance to the EAC. This condition is very painful and can be overlooked when the ear speculum is introduced. The condition will not improve without an incision and removal of the pus

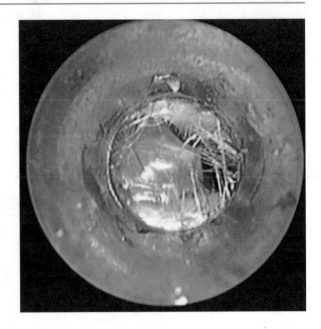

A drainage should be performed with the scalpel with local or surface anaesthesia. It is possible to overlook the furuncle when inserting the ear speculum into the EAC.

Chronic external otitis often develops in patients with seborrheic dermatitis, diabetes, hypersensitivity to soap and shampoo, or chronic otitis media [15]. Therapy of chronic external otitis needs persistence. Patients have to protect the EAC from water. Local therapy with drops that lower the pH in the EAC is also recommendable.

3.10.1 Benign Necrotizing External Otitis

Benign necrotizing external otitis is a rare condition of unknown aetiology characterised by ulceration on the EAC floor where it overlays an area of bony necrosis. It is probably caused by compromised vascular supply. It is very important to distinguish the condition from necrotizing otitis externa or carcinoma of the EAC, because treatment differs significantly. In benign necrotizing otitis externa, long term medical treatment is advocated. Surgery is very seldom needed and is usually successful (Figs. 3.51 and 3.52).

3.10.2 Necrotizing (Malignant) External Otitis

Necrotizing external otitis develops in patients with diabetes, immunocompromised patients especially after organ transplantations, or during or after chemotherapy as a complication of acute external otitis. It is caused by *Pseudomonas aeruginosa* and

Fig. 3.51 Left ear. Benign necrotizing otitis externa is a rare finding in the EAC and is characterised by skin defect mostly on the floor of the EAC and exposed necrotic bone. On the picture the skin defect is already healing on the floor of the EAC, on the anterior wall a crust is covering the skin defect

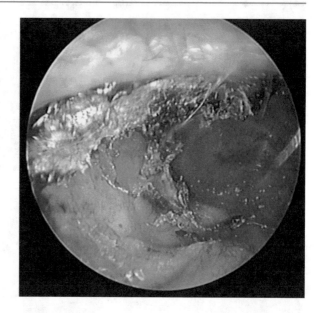

Fig. 3.52 Left ear. Same patient as in the previous figure. The skin defect healed after time. Part of the bone on the EAC floor was necrotic, leaving the defect

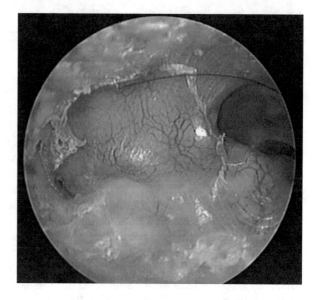

is characterised by osteomyelitis which spreads in the lateral skull base with possible involvement of the cranial nerves.

The main symptoms are pain, foetid secretion from the EAC, granulations in the EAC, and malfunction of cranial nerves, especially the facial nerve. During clinical examination patients should also be tested for meningeal signs.

In the EAC granulations with exposed bone can be observed (Fig. 3.53) Usually blood sugar and HbA1c levels are high. A high-resolution CT scan should be

Fig. 3.53 Left ear.
Necrotizing external otitis
in elderly diabetic patient.
The patient had
granulations in the anterior
wall of the EAC. These
were removed and the
abscess was cleaned with a
curette. A skin defect is
still visible, but the
patient's condition is
improving

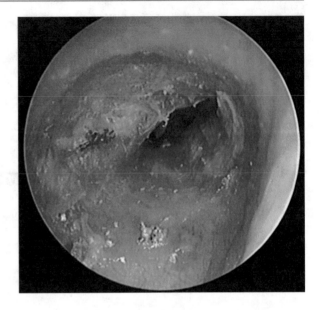

performed to see the extent of osteomyelitis. Therapy consists of curettage of the granulation tissue, correcting the levels of blood sugar and long-term antibiotic therapy against Pseudomonas (at least 6 weeks).

3.11   Tumours of the External Ear Canal

Benign neoplasm of the EAC are rare and usually arise from ceruminous glands. They appear in the cartilaginous portion of the EAC (Figs. 3.54, 3.55, 3.56, 3.57, and 3.58). The most common are ceruminous adenoma and pleomorphic adenoma. Biopsies should be taken with margin of normal tissue to rule out the invasion of the tumour into surrounding tissue. The treatment is local excision.

Malignant tumours are also rare (Figs. 3.59 and 3.60). Of these the squamous cell carcinoma is the most common malignancy (Fig. 3.61). Adenoid cystic carcinoma and acinic cell carcinoma can also be found. Patients have otorrhea, pain, and hearing loss. Symptoms may mimic chronic otitis externa or media. During otoscopy a tumour is difficult to distinguish from granulation tissue. Diagnosis is confirmed by biopsy which must be repeated even under general anaesthesia, if the result is negative. Usually both CT and MRI scans are needed. Treatment is multidisciplinary including otologist, oncologist and sometimes also a plastic reconstructive surgeon.

Fig. 3.54 Left ear. On the anterior wall of the EAC meatus a tumour with a rough surface with no ulceration can be seen. The patient is an elderly woman, who observed the condition for many months. Histology showed that the tumour was seborrheic keratosis. Beside histologic verification, no other treatment is needed

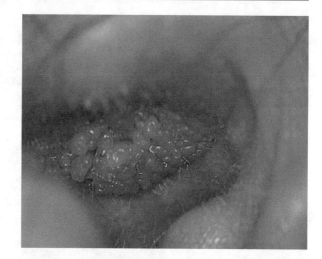

Fig. 3.55 Right ear. A tumour on the anterior EAC wall covered with intact skin. Histologically it proved to be an intravascular papillary endothelial hyperplasia (IPEH), also known as Masson's tumour. It is a rare vascular lesion. Symptoms are associated with compressive effects on adjacent structures

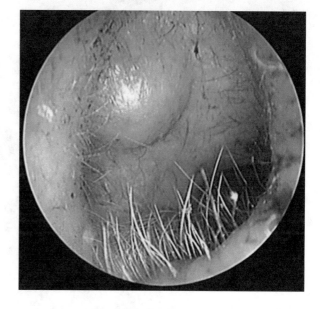

Fig. 3.56 Right ear.
Fibroma of the EAC in the
middle third on the
superior canal wall. Note
the limited extent of the
lesion without necrosis and
inflammation. Intact skin
covers the tumour

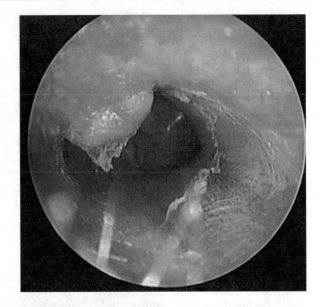

Fig. 3.57 Right ear.
Chondroma of the
EAC. The posterosuperior
part of the EAC is
occupied with a round
lesion that partially
obstructs the
EAC. Histology showed
that it was a chondroma

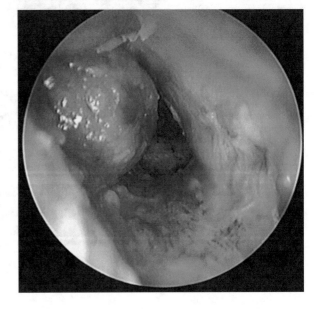

Fig. 3.58 Left ear. A polyp completely obstructing the medial third of the EAC. Its origin may be inflammatory or tumorous. A biopsy and imaging are always necessary before starting the treatment

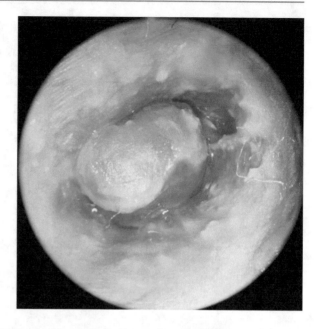

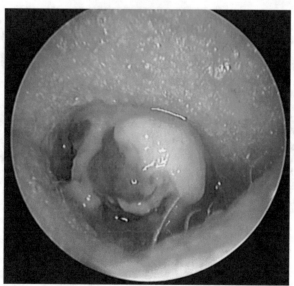

Fig. 3.59 Left ear. Adenocarcinoma of the endolymphatic saccus. On the posterior wall of the EAC a tumorous mass is visible obstructing almost the entire lumen of the EAC. Around the tumour a part of necrotic white tissue is visible, with some discharge in the medial part of the EAC. The patient was an elderly lady who had problems with her left ear for a long time and could not come to a decision about treatment. The tumour grew from the endolymphatic sac through the mastoid and finally through the posterior wall of the EAC. Eventually it was the facial paralysis that made her visit a doctor. In cases with this kind of otoscopic findings, imaging (CT and MRI) of the temporal bone and a biopsy should be performed

Fig. 3.60 Right ear. A scar following tumour excision is visible in the posterior wall. The tumour was a basocellular carcinoma, which was not excised completely in another institution. During reexcision it was found the tumour had spread subcutaneously to the middle part of the EAC. Histologic verification of tumour margins is very important

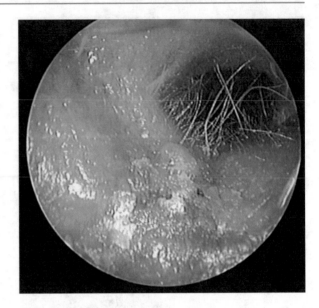

Fig. 3.61 Right ear. A tumour in the medial and middle part of the EAC covered with pus. The patient was first treated with conservative therapy for chronic otitis media with no effect. A biopsy revealed a squamous cell carcinoma. The patient was treated with subtotal petrosectomy including the obliteration of the EAC followed by radiotherapy and resulting in a disease-free period of 10 years

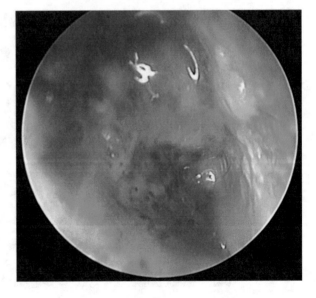

References

1. Kim GW, Park JH, Kwon OJ, Kim DH, Kim CW. Clinical characteristics of epidermoid cysts of the external auditory canal. J Audiol Otol. 2016;20(1):36–40.
2. Turetsky DB, Vines FS, Clayman DA. Surfer's ear: exostoses of the external ear canal. Am J Neuroradiol. 1990;11(6):1217–8.
3. Thompson SK, Wein RO, Dutcher PO. External auditory canal foreign body removal; management practices and outcomes. Laryngoscope. 2003;113(11):1912–5.
4. Tiago RSL, Salgado DC, Correa JP, Pio MRB, Lambert EE. Foreign body in ear, nose and oropharynx: experience from tertiary hospital. Braz J Otorhinolaryngol. 2006;72(2):177–81.
5. Schulze SL, Kerschner J, Beste D. Pediatric external auditory canal foreign bodies: a review of 698 cases. Otolaryngol Head Neck Surg. 2002;127:73–8.
6. Kotikoski MJ, Palmu AA, Nokso-Koivisto J, Kleemola M. Evaluation of the role of respiratory viruses in acute myringitis in children less than two years of age. Pediatr Infect Dis J. 2002;21(7):636–41.
7. Hariri MA. Sensorineural hearing loss in bullous myringitis. A prospective study of eighteen patients. Clin Otolaryngol Allied Sci. 1990;15:351–3.
8. Stoney P, Kwok P, Hawke M. Granular myringitis: a review. J Otolaryngol. 1992;21(2):129–35.
9. Moser G, Emberger M, Tóth M, Roesch S, Rasp G, Laimer M. Ectopic apocrine glands as a predisposing factor for postinflammatory medial meatal fibrosis. Otol Neurotol. 2015;36(1):191–7.
10. Sharon JD, Khwaja SS, Drescher A, Gay H, Chole RA. Osteoradionecrosis of the temporal bone. Otol Neurotol. 2014;35(7):1207–17.
11. Morgan M, Nathwani D. Facial nerve palsy and infection: the unfolding story. Clin Infect Dis. 1992;14:263–71.
12. Gondikar S, Parikh V, Parikh R. Herpes zoster oticus: a rare clinical entity. Contemp Clin Dent. 2010;1(2):127–9.
13. Kinishi M, Amatsu M, Mohri M, Saito M, Hasegawa T, Hasegawa S. Acyclovir improves recovery rate of facial nerve palsy in Ramsay Hunt syndrome. Aurus Nasus Larynx. 2001;28:223–6.
14. Ho T, Vrabec JT, Yoo D, Coker NJ. Otomycosis: clinical features and treatment implications. Otolaryngol Head Neck Surg. 2006;135(5):787–91.
15. Simon F. Diagnosis and treatment of external otitis. HNO. 2020;68(11):881–8.

Secretory Otitis Media

4

In secretory otitis media (SOM), a transudate (technically an exudate) forms in the middle ear. The eardrum is intact but immobile, due to the fluid inside of the middle ear. Fluid inside of the middle ear can be serous or mucoid (Figs. 4.1, 4.2, 4.3, 4.4, 4.5, 4.6, and 4.7), depending also on the duration of the SOM.

Early diagnosis of SOM in children is very important. The condition may affect language acquisition and increases the risk of learning difficulties [1].

SOM can be divided into three stages:

− The *initial stage*, the period from the first pathological action on the middle ear mucosa to the beginning of accumulation of fluid in the middle ear.

Fig. 4.1 Right ear. A dark yellow effusion can be identified in the middle ear. Note the incipient thinning and retraction of the drum in the posteroinferior quarter

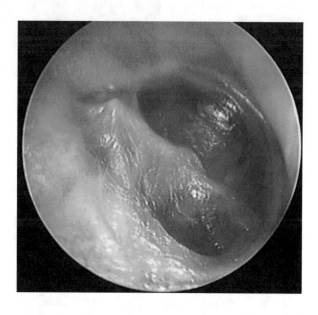

© The Author(s), under exclusive license to Springer Nature Switzerland AG 2022
J. Rebol, *Otoscopy Findings*, https://doi.org/10.1007/978-3-031-03979-9_4

Fig. 4.2 Right ear. Serous effusion inside of the middle ear with the air bubbles in the anterior part of the middle ear

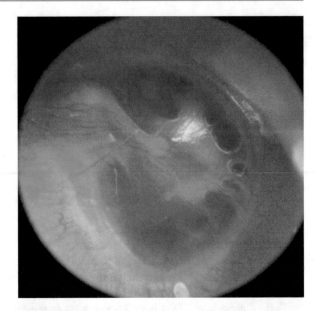

Fig. 4.3 Right ear. Myringosclerosis in the posterior quadrants of the eardrum and anteriorly in front of the annulus. Brown fluid in the middle ear can be seen through the eardrum in the anterosuperior quadrant. The patient had previously had a tympanic tube insertion that resulted in myringosclerosis

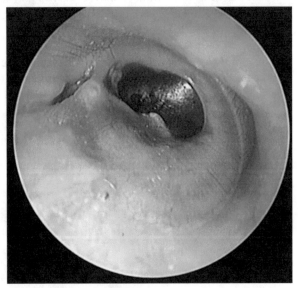

– The *secretory stage*, the period of effusion, accumulation of fluid in the middle ear. This may last from a few months to several years.
– The *degenerative stage* when the effusion abates.

In the initial stage the mucosa of the middle ear transforms into secretory mucosa with the formation of pathological mucous glands. Basal cells differentiate into goblet cells and ciliated cells. Through further intense division of the basal cells,

Fig. 4.4 Right ear. The
eardrum has an opaque
appearance because of the
thick secretion inside of
the middle ear. At
myringotomy the fluid was
thick, glue-like, and such a
condition can also be
called *glue ear*

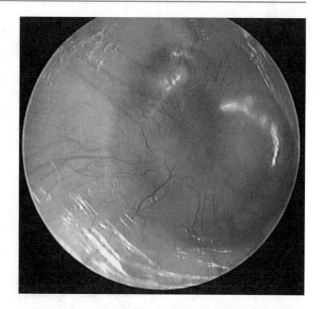

Fig. 4.5 Right ear. The
eardrum is retracted and
opaque due to thick fluid in
the middle ear

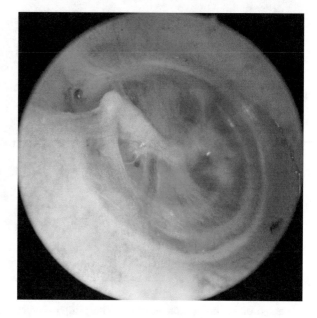

they form cylinders that grow deeper and divide dichotomously into two or several
tubules. During the degeneration process, the lumen of the glands becomes filled
with mucus, dilating the duct system; the secretory epithelium is widespread and
gradually transformed into nonsecretory epithelium [2].

The position of the tympanic membrane is a key for differentiating acute otitis
media (AOM) and otitis media with effusion. In acute otitis media, the tympanic
membrane is usually bulging outwards. In otitis media with effusion, it is typically

Fig. 4.6 Right ear. The eardrum is opaque, due to mucoid secretion in the middle ear. The eardrum is thick and mostly in the neutral position, apart from the anterosuperior quadrant, where a mild retraction is present

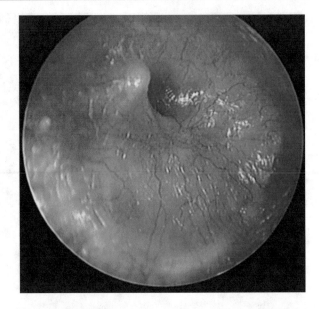

Fig. 4.7 Left ear. The eardrum is opaque, thick, and bulged in the posterior quadrants. Secretion in the middle ear is mucoid and partly suppurative due to an infection of the middle ear

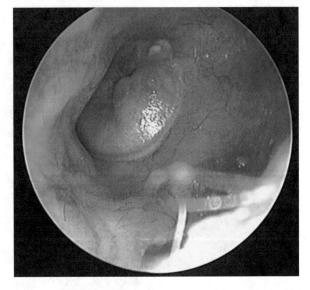

retracted or in the neutral position. The tympanic membrane can be thickened in both acute otitis media and otitis media with effusion, thereby reducing its transparency. A yellow or grey middle ear effusion can be seen behind the tympanic membrane in either condition. In cases of mucoid effusion, the drum usually loses its translucency, becoming opaque, a grey-white, dull colour, and thick in texture [3].

Sometimes we see air bubbles, especially in the anterior part of the middle ear (Figs. 4.8, 4.9, 4.10, 4.11, and 4.12). Usually this is a good prognostic sign,

Fig. 4.8 Right ear. The eardrum is in a neutral position, there are many air bubbles in the middle ear. When the patient performed autoinsufflation, the air bubbles in the middle ear moved back and forth

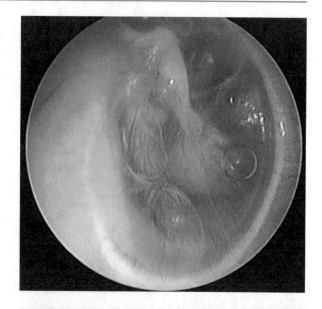

Fig. 4.9 Right ear. Air bubbles in the anterior part of the middle ear. The eardrum is transparent. Fluid in the remaining part of the middle ear is yellow brown

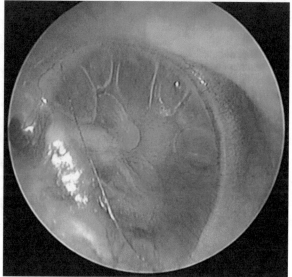

indicating that the ventilation of the middle ear is once again functioning. The appearance of bubbles can also sometimes be seen under the microscope during autoinflation when a patient performs the Valsalva manoeuvre. Sometimes we can also see the level of the fluid in the middle ear (Figs. 4.13 and 4.14). The eardrum can be retracted, even developing retraction pockets (Figs. 4.15 and 4.16).

SOM arises as a consequence of Eustachian tube obstruction, which can be caused by enlarged adenoids (the most common cause in children), allergies,

Fig. 4.10 Right ear. The eardrum is in a neutral position. A crust is located on the posterior part. Underneath the eardrum in the anterosuperior quadrant an air bubble can be identified (arrow). A light reflex in the anteroinferior quadrant can also be observed even though the middle ear condition is not normal

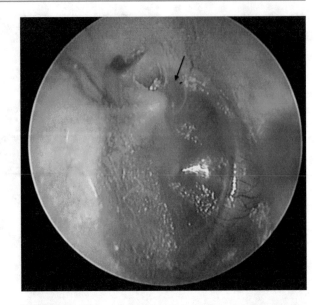

Fig. 4.11 Left ear. A single air bubble can be seen under the posterosuperior quadrant of the eardrum with effusion in the remaining part of the middle ear

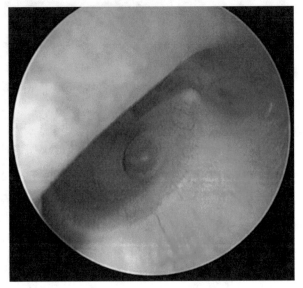

infections, or tumour in the nasopharynx. In cases of unilateral SOM in adult patients we must exclude the possibility of a tumour in the nasopharynx. SOM can also be caused by a malfunctioning of the muscles which open the Eustachian tube. This is a very common finding in patients with cheilognatopalatoschisis. Irregularity in Eustachian tube function can also be seen in certain syndromes such as Down syndrome.

Fig. 4.12 Left ear. Serous effusion in the middle ear. Large air bubbles can be seen under all quadrants of the eardrum. A retraction pocket is present in the posterosuperior quadrant, which is adherent to the long process of the incus—*myringoincudopexy*

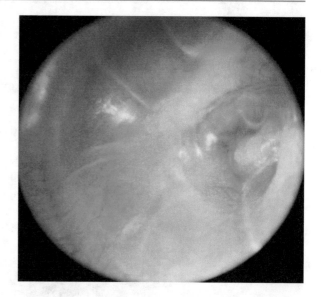

Fig. 4.13 Right ear. Four air bubbles can be seen in the anterosuperior quadrant with effusion in the remaining part of the middle ear. This is denser at the bottom, where it appears brown and forms a distinct layer

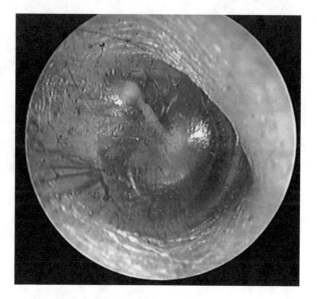

Occlusion of the Eustachian tube leads to negative pressure in the middle ear, that is caused by resorption of oxygen in the mucosa of the middle ear. It results in fluid transudation into the middle ear. Postinflammatory alterations in the middle ear mucosa and Eustachian tube lead to goblet cell metaplasia and hypersecretion that cause the persistence of the effusion.

Diagnosis is set by otoscopy and tympanometry, where, in the presence of fluid in the middle ear, the eardrum is immobile (type B tympanogram), and by audiometry, revealing conductive hearing loss.

Fig. 4.14 Left ear. A level
of mucoid fluid can be
seen in the inferior
quadrants of the eardrum.
The remaining part of the
middle ear is filled with air.
A follow-up of the patient
is needed in about a month
by when the fluid will
probably have resolved

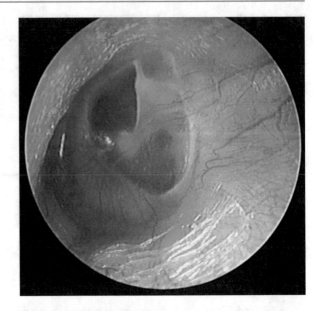

Fig. 4.15 Left ear. An
opaque eardrum in the
normal position. The fluid
in the middle ear is
mucoid. The patient had
recurrent SOM. A
tympanic tube was already
inserted formerly in the
anteroinferior quadrant,
where a small retraction
pocket is visible

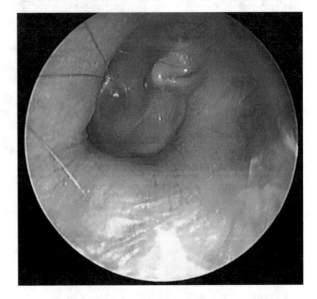

If the secretory otitis persists for more than 3 months on both sides, an adenotomy and myringotomy with insertion of tympanostomy tubes (TT) (Figs. 4.17,
4.18, and 4.19) should be performed. Insertion of tympanostomy tubes is the most
common operation in children. Because of the recurrence of SOM, many children
undergo the procedure several times.

Patients with tympanostomy tubes (TT) should avoid water due to the possibility
of developing acute otitis media. The shape of TT differs depending on how long the

Fig. 4.16 Right ear. The eardrum is retracted with yellow effusion in the middle ear. The patient had long-term Eustachian tube dysfunction. The eardrum is adherent to the head of stapes, the lenticular process of the incus is resorbed. Such a condition is called *myringostapediopexy*

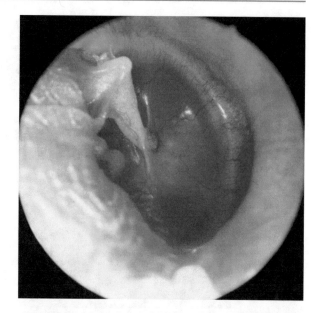

Fig. 4.17 Right ear. On the posterior wall of the EAC, epithelial scabs can be seen. The eardrum is in a normal position but is opaque due to mucoid effusion. A titanium TT was inserted in the anterosuperior quadrant but is already extruded and the eardrum underneath has healed up. Due to the occlusion of the Eustachian tube, SOM developed again

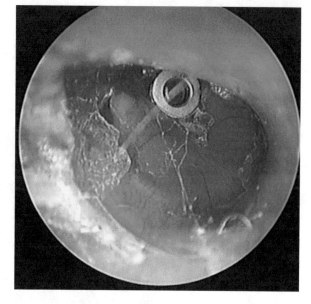

TT should remain in place. TTs are usually left in place for 6 months, then they are extruded, and the eardrum heals. It has been found that only 36–43% of patients could be considered completely cured, having normal hearing and normal tubal function, 1–5 years after grommet insertion [4]. A temporary improvement in hearing reduces the risk of delayed speech and language development. Changes in the eardrum such as myringosclerosis and atrophy can sometimes also be observed [5].

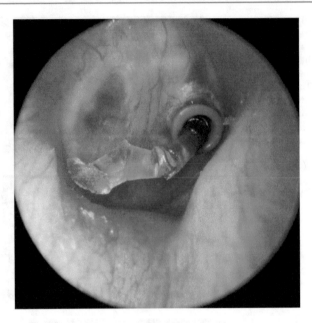

Fig. 4.18 Right ear. Small exostosis on the anterior wall of the EAC. A durable tympanic tube which has a larger diameter was inserted in the anterosuperior quadrant. The patient has aspirin exacerbated respiratory disease (AERD) also known as Samter's Triad, characterised by nasal polyps, asthma, and aspirin intolerance. Beside these symptoms, patients with this disease often have secretory otitis due to the changes in the mucosa in the middle ear and nasal cavity (common respiratory mucosa). Despite the TT, the mucosa still produces the secretion, which can be seen as a scab inside the lumen of the TT and extending beyond the tube

Fig. 4.19 Left ear. A durable TT was inserted in the anterosuperior quadrant of the eardrum. The middle ear became inflamed, a red polyp can be seen in the lumen of the TT (as an expression of the chronic irritation). In most cases local antibiotic drops are sufficient to heal the inflammation

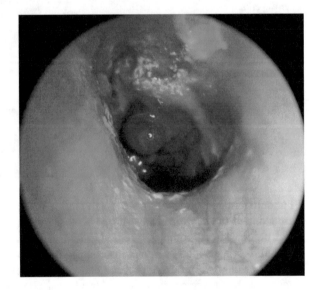

Fig. 4.20 Left ear. An extruded durable TT with some epithelial scabs on the posterior wall of the EAC. The TT has a small wire by which it can be pulled out of the EAC

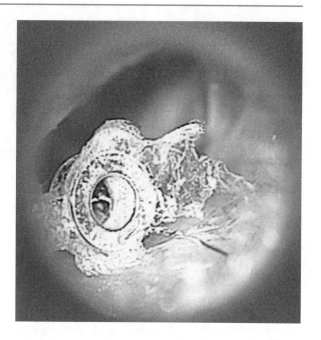

In patients with chronic secretory otitis, long-term TTs can be inserted. These can stay in place for a year or even longer (Fig. 4.20). They have a deeper hollow in the middle ear and some have wings (T-Tube) that prevent the extrusion of the tube (Fig. 4.21).

After TT insertion patients have to be followed up and the TTs should be removed when they extrude. After TT extrusion, the integrity of the eardrum should be checked. In cases where a small perforation persists, this can be closed with a fat graft myringoplasty.

To inflate the middle ear, various methods have been used, including the Valsalva manoeuvre and passive inflation with the Politzer test. With children it is also possible to teach them to perform autoinflation using a specially designed nose tube with a balloon attached to it [6].

Chronic recurrent SOM is characterised by a history of several courses of TT insertions. In such patients, beside TT placement, a balloon dilatation of the Eustachian tube can be performed with good results [7].

Fig. 4.21 Right ear. The patient had a skull base fracture many years ago. Ever since, her Eustachian tube does not work properly resulting in chronic secretory otitis. A long-term T-shaped tube was placed in her middle ear and will stay in place for a number of years

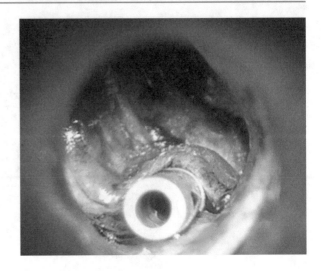

References

1. Pichichero ME. Acute otitis media: Part I. Improving diagnostic accuracy. Am Fam Physician. 2000;61(7):2051–6.
2. Tos M. Pathogenesis and pathology of chronic secretory otitis media. Ann Otol Rhinol Laryngol Suppl. 1980;89:91–7.
3. Sade J, Luntz M, Pitashny R. Diagnosis and treatment of secretory otitis media. Otolaryngol Clin North Am. 1989;22(1):1–14.
4. Tos M, Poulsen G. Secretory otitis media. Late results of treatment with grommets. Arch Otolaryngol. 1976;102(11):672–5.
5. Caye-Thomasen P, Stengerup SE, Jørgensen G, Drozdiziewic D, Bonding P, Tos M. Myringotomy versus ventilation tubes in secretory otitis media: eardrum pathology, hearing and eustachian tube function 25 years after treatment. Otol Neurotol. 2008;29(5):649–57.
6. Stangerup SE, Sederberg-Olsen J, Balle V. Autoinflation as a treatment of secretory otitis media. A randomized controlled study. Arch Otolaryngol Head Neck Surg. 1992;18(2):149–52.
7. Li YQ, Chen YB, Yin GD, Zeng XL. Effect of balloon dilation eustachian tuboplasty combined with tympanic tube insertion in the treatment of chronic recurrent secretory otitis media. Eur Arch Otorhinolaryngol. 2019;276(10):2715–20.

Adhesive Otitis

5

In adhesive otitis media adhesions form between an atrophic and retracted eardrum and the medial wall of the middle ear [1]. Retraction of the eardrum, either of the pars tensa or the pars flaccida, is assumed to be a pathological route, leading to middle ear and attic cholesteatoma. The aetiology of retractions is complex, but chronic negative middle ear pressure is the major cause. Over time necrosis of the long process of the incus and stapes suprastructure can also occur. If the eardrum is adherent to the incus, we talk of *myringoincudopexy*. In incus necrosis the eardrum is adherent to the stapes and is called *myringostapediopexy*. Patients with eardrum retraction and atelectasis can raise the eardrum with autoinflation manoeuvres such as Valsalva or Toynbee. In advanced adhesive otitis (type IV in the Sadé classification) this is no longer possible. The condition is irreversible because histologic examination showed that in adhesive otitis the lamina propria of the atrophic eardrum is very thin or absent.

Retraction of the eardrum is caused by constant negative pressure in the middle ear due to Eustachian tube dysfunction. Adhesions between the eardrum and the middle ear mucosa are probably caused by an episode of suppurative otitis during the course of disease. Larger retraction pockets may collect migrating epithelium and can later develop a cholesteatoma.

According to the Sadé classification [2] we can distinguish the following stages of pars tensa retractions:

1. slight eardrum retraction (Figs. 5.1, 5.2, 5.3, 5.4, and 5.5);
2. a retracted eardrum gets in touch with incus or stapes (Figs. 5.6, 5.7, 5.8, 5.9, 5.10, 5.11, 5.12, and 5.13);
3. a retracted eardrum is touching the promontory (Figs. 5.14, 5.15, and 5.16);
4. adhesive otitis—eardrum is attached to the promontory (Figs. 5.17 and 5.18);
5. spontaneous perforation in the atelectatic eardrum with suppuration and formation of polyps. This usually occurs in atelectasis stage III or IV (Figs. 5.19, 5.20, 5.21, 5.22, 5.23, and 5.24).

© The Author(s), under exclusive license to Springer Nature Switzerland AG 2022
J. Rebol, *Otoscopy Findings*, https://doi.org/10.1007/978-3-031-03979-9_5

Fig. 5.1 Left ear. Atrophic and slightly retracted eardrum (stage I of Sadé classification of pars tensa retractions)

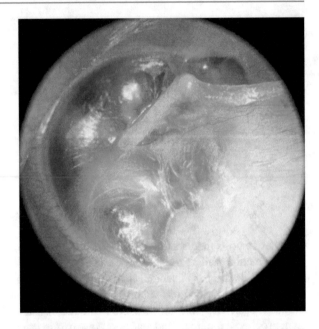

Fig. 5.2 Right ear. The eardrum is atrophic in the posterior quadrants. When performing the autoinflation Valsalva manoeuvre, the eardrum bulges beyond its normal position

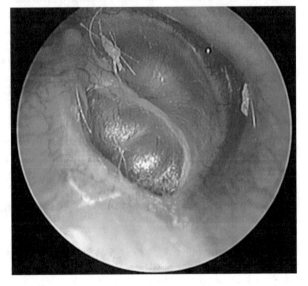

Fig. 5.3 Left ear. An atrophic and bulged eardrum in the posterior part during autoinflation

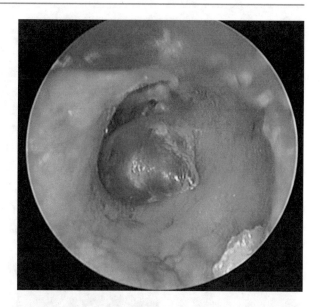

Fig. 5.4 Left ear. Another example of a bulged eardrum at autoinflation. The patient had a sensation of fullness in the ear with diminished hearing and often performed the Valsalva manoeuvre trying to improve his hearing. He was made aware that the bulla of an atrophic eardrum could perforate after repeated autoinflation manoeuvres

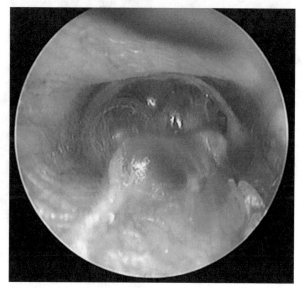

Fig. 5.5 Left ear. The eardrum is atrophic and retracted in the anterosuperior quadrant. Stage I of Sadé classification. The retraction extends towards the ostium of the Eustachian tube

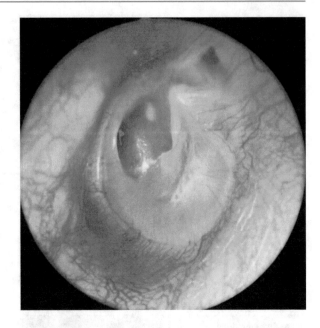

Fig. 5.6 Right ear. Retraction of the eardrum in the central part. Through the retracted eardrum an effusion and an air bubble in the anterosuperior quadrant in the middle ear can be seen. The eardrum is also in contact with the long process of the incus—myringoincudopexy

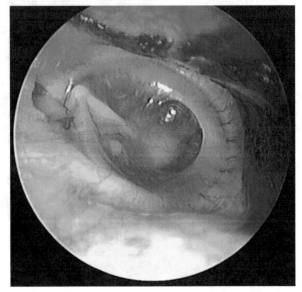

Fig. 5.7 Left ear. Retraction of the eardrum in the superior part. A white plaque is visible in the inferior part—myringosclerosis. The eardrum is adherent to the incus and stapes—*myringo incudostapediopexy*

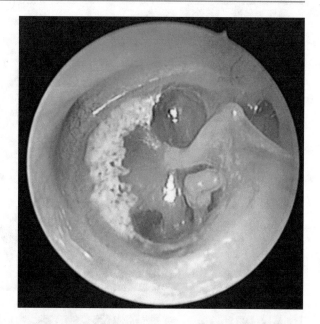

Fig. 5.8 Left ear. The entire eardrum is retracted with the air bubbles in the middle ear. The eardrum is adherent to the long process of the incus—myringoincudopexy

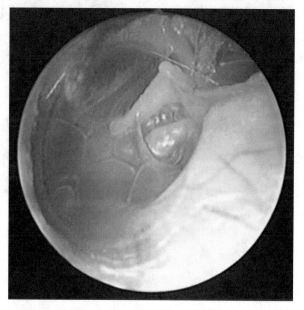

Fig. 5.9 Right ear. A
situation similar to the
previous figure. The
eardrum is mainly retracted
in the posterior part with
myringoincudopexy.
Granulation tissue at the
annulus, the retraction
pocket shows no
inflammation

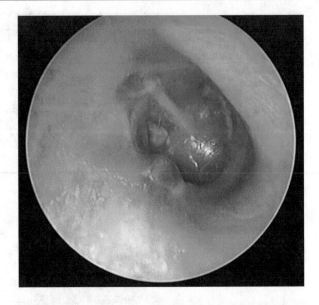

Fig. 5.10 Left ear. The
retraction pocket is limited
to the posterosuperior
quadrant of the eardrum.
The bottom of the
retraction pocket is not
completely visible but
seems to be dry. The long
process of the incus is still
present—
myringoincudopexy

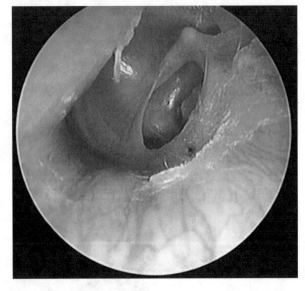

Fig. 5.11 Left ear. Retraction pocket in the posterosuperior quadrant of the eardrum, the retraction also extends to the attic. The long process of the incus is completely resorbed—*myringostapediopexy*. The pars flaccida of the eardrum is also maximally retracted (Tos classification type II)

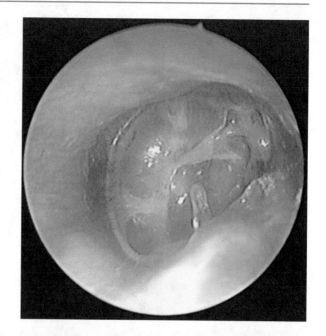

Fig. 5.12 Right ear. A dry retraction pocket in the posterior quadrants of the eardrum. The long process of the incus and the suprastructure of the stapes are absent

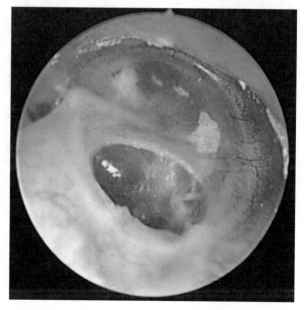

Fig. 5.13 Left ear. Retraction pocket in the posterosuperior quadrant of the eardrum which also extends to the attic. *M* malleus, *CI* corpus of the incus, *LI* long process of the incus, *F* facial nerve, *HS* head of the stapes, *SM* stapedial muscle

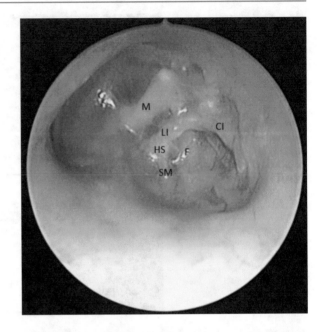

Fig. 5.14 Left ear. The eardrum is adherent to the promontory in the medial wall in the posterior part of the middle ear. There is some fluid in the anterior part of the middle ear. In the posterior part myringostapediopexy is present, the distal part of the long process of the incus is resorbed (Sadé stage 3). *M* malleus, *LI* long process of the incus, *OW* oval window, *P* promontory, *RW* round window

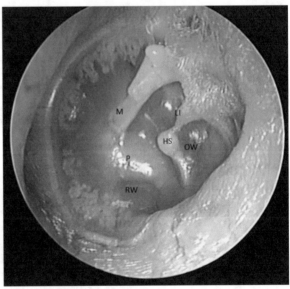

Even when proposing this classification, Sadé noted that the classification of retraction pockets is arbitrary and that intermediary stages do exist. From 1976 to 2007, 12 different staging systems have been described for tympanic membrane retractions, among them classifications from Charachon, Dornhoffer, Borgstein, and Tran Ba Huy which also refer to the visibility of the bottom of the retraction

Fig. 5.15 Left ear. Adhesion of the eardrum to the promontory in the posterior quadrants of the eardrum. The long process of the incus is resorbed, myringostapediopexy is present. In the anterior quadrants myringosclerosis is present, which prevented the eardrum from thinning and retracting (Sadé stage 3)

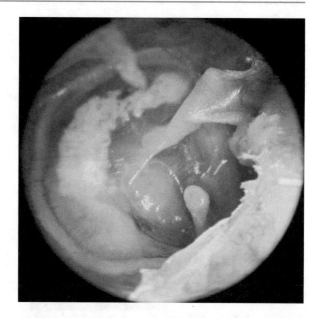

Fig. 5.16 Left ear. Adhesion mostly in the superior part of the middle ear, the malleus handle is medialised, ossicles still appear intact

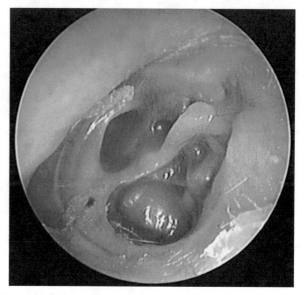

Fig. 5.17 Right ear. The eardrum is completely adherent to the medial wall of the middle ear. The long process of the incus was resorbed, myringostapediopexy is present (Sadé stage 4). The tympanic ostium of the Eustachian tube can be seen through the eardrum in the anteroinferior quadrant

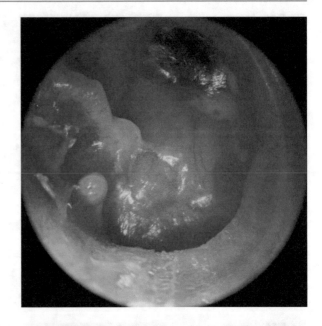

Fig. 5.18 Left ear. Adhesion of the eardrum on the promontory, ossicles are still intact (Sadé stage 4)

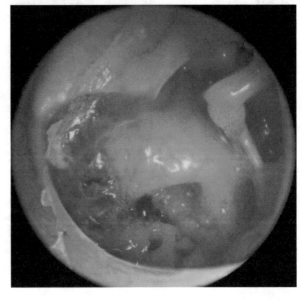

Fig. 5.19 Left ear. Retraction pocket in the posterior part of the middle ear. Auditory ossicles are still intact. The bottom of the retraction pocket is not visible but there appears to be a perforation because of epithelial layer emerging from the retraction pocket (Sadé stage 4). A retraction pocket is also present in the attic

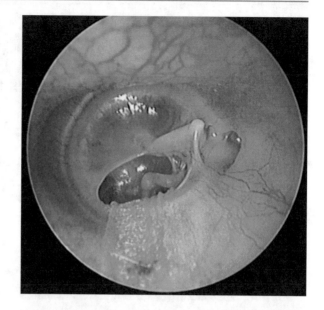

Fig. 5.20 Right ear. Another example of adhesive otitis stage 5 according to Sadé. A large retraction pocket in the posterior part of the middle ear extends to the posterior attic. The long process of the incus and the suprastructure of the stapes are resorbed. There is granulation tissue in the oval niche

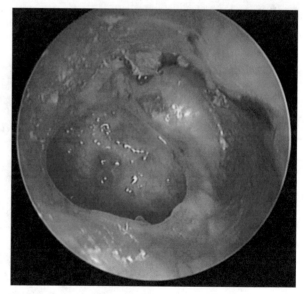

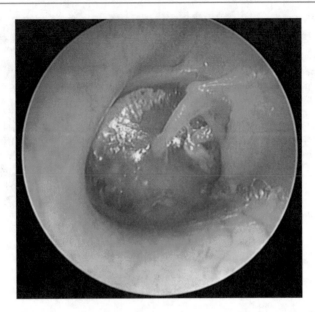

Fig. 5.21 Left ear. Myringoincudostapedopexy, the retraction pocket is not clearly visible but, based on the epithelial line coming out of the retraction pocket, there appears to be a perforation (Sadé stage 5)

Fig. 5.22 Right ear. Adhesion of the eardrum to the medial wall of the middle ear with suppuration and some dry scabs in the retraction pockets (Sadé stage 5)

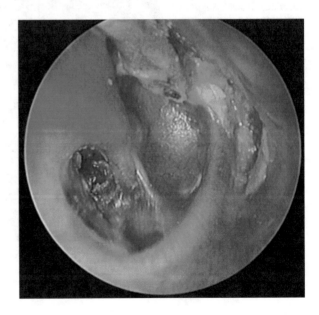

Fig. 5.23 Right ear. Final stage of adhesive otitis: the eardrum is adherent to the medial wall of the middle ear. The handle of malleus is also adherent to the medial wall. The ear is wet, probably due to inflammation in parts of the retraction that is not visible

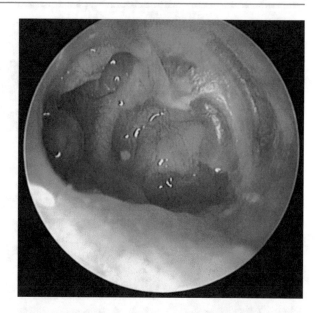

Fig. 5.24 Right ear. Another example of the final stage of adhesive otitis. A complete atelectasis of the eardrum, resorbed incus, and stapes suprastructure. Suppuration is also present, with desiccated secretions in the superior part of the middle ear and the attic

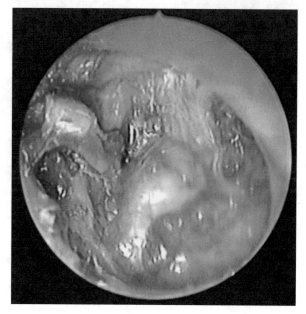

pocket and keratin accumulation in the retraction pocket (Figs. 5.25, 5.26, 5.27, 5.28, and 5.29) [3].

The treatment of adhesive otitis or tympanic membrane retractions depends on the degree of retraction, hearing loss, and the patient's requirements. In moderate degrees of retraction (stages 1–2), regular follow-up of patients is sensible. Patients with keratin accumulation and otorrhea are candidates for surgical repair.

Fig. 5.25 Left ear. Beside the pars tensa retraction pocket in the posterior part of the middle ear, there is also a small dimple in the attic (Tos type I). The lateral attic wall or *scutum* is not eroded

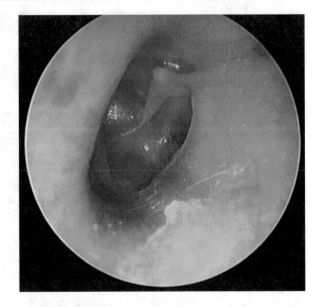

Fig. 5.26 Right ear. Beside the pars tensa retraction stage 2 with myringoincudopexy, there is also a retraction pocket in the attic. Part of the lateral wall is eroded (Tos type III)

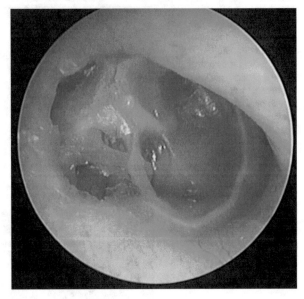

Long-term tympanostomy tubes (TT) could be also applied, ordinary TTs are unable to prevent the final condition in the long run of the disease. Good results were reported with sub-annular placement of TTs (Fig. 4.21) [4]. Grade 2 and 3 retraction pockets can be excised transmeatally with simultaneous placement of TTs [5].

If the long process of the incus or even the stapes suprastructure are missing, tympanoplasty with cartilage and ossiculoplasty is indicated. An air-bone gap >20 dB could be an indication for retraction pocket surgery. With the introduction

Fig. 5.27 Left ear. Defect in the attic. The head of the malleus is partly resorbed. The upper part of the retraction is not visible (Tos type IV)

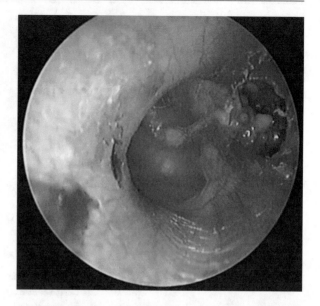

Fig. 5.28 Right ear. A large attic defect, the head of the malleus and the body of the incus are absent. Keratin is accumulated in the bottom of the pocket, but it is not possible to see its extent (Tos type IV)

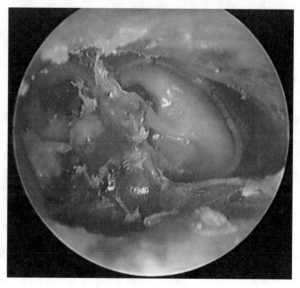

of cartilage as a material for tympanic membrane reconstruction, the results of the operations improved significantly in regard to recurrent retractions. The results can be improved with simultaneous Eustachian tube balloon dilatation [6].

Pars flaccida retractions were classified by Tos. According to his classification type I represents small attic dimple, type II maximally retracted pars flaccida, draped over the neck of the malleus, type III as type II with erosion of lateral attic wall, and type IV for cases of deep retraction with unreachable accumulated keratin [7].

Fig. 5.29 Left ear. Accidental finding. A large defect in the attic can be seen with complete absence of the incus. The patient was never operated but had otitis in the childhood. The evacuated cavity is clean. When such a condition occurs it is called a spontaneous atticotomy

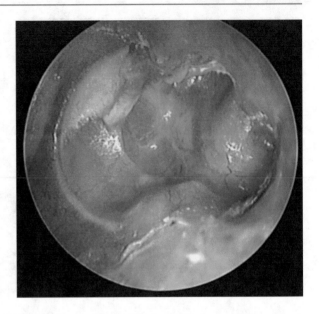

The staging systems from Sadé and Tos depend on how far the retraction has progressed medially and whether there is an involvement of other middle ear structures. Although both systems are well designed and have been in use for many years, it was found that clinicians sometimes have problems in applying them to clinical situations [8].

References

1. Cawthorne T. Chronic adhesive otitis. J Laryngol Otol. 1956;70(10):559–64.
2. Sadé J, Avraham S, Brown M. Atelectasis, retraction pockets and cholesteatoma. Acta Otolaryngol. 1981;92(5–6):501–12.
3. Alzahrani M, Saliba I. Tympanic membrane retraction pocket staging: is it worthwhile? Eur Arch Otorhinolaryngol. 2014;271(6):1361–8.
4. Ciodaro F, Cammaroto G, Galletti B, Galletti F. Subannular T-tubes for the treatment of adhesive otitis media. B-ENT. 2016;12(2):131–5.
5. Ráth G, Gerlinger I, Csákányi Z, Sultész M, Gaál V, Katona G. Transmeatal excision of pars tensa retraction pockets with simultaneous ventilation tube insertion in children: a prospective study. Eur Arch Otorhinolaryngol. 2011;268(11):1549–56.
6. Si Y, Chen Y, Xu G, Chen X, He W, Zhang Z. Cartilage tympanoplasty combined with eustachian tube balloon dilatation in the treatment of adhesive otitis media. Laryngoscope. 2019;129(6):1462–7.
7. Tos M, Poulsen G. Attic retractions following secretory otitis. Acta Otolaryngol. 1980;89(5–6):479–86.
8. Pothier DD. The Sadé and Tos staging systems: not adequately reliable methods of staging retraction of tympanic membrane? Clin Otolaryngol. 2009;34(5):506–7.

Acute and Chronic Otitis

6

Treating otitis media is the most frequent reason for visiting a paediatrician and the most frequent cause for prescribing antibiotics to children. It is estimated that a child in developed countries spends an average of 6–7 weeks on antibiotics by the age of 2. In an urban environment around 90% of children have suffered from AOM.

Most AOM happens in childhood, though it can also occur in adulthood. Myringotomy has an important place in the treatment of otitis media and is also the most frequent operation under general anaesthesia in the USA. Otitis media is also considered one of the manifestations or associated symptoms of COVID-19 [1].

6.1   Definition

Otitis media (OM) is an inflammatory condition in the middle ear, related to effusion behind the eardrum. It is connected to upper respiratory tract infections and dysfunction of the Eustachian tube.

Otitis media can be further classified with regard to the type of fluid in the middle ear: serous, mucoid, and suppurative. Clinically OM can be divided into secretory otitis, AOM, and chronic suppurative otitis media (CSOM). CSOM occurs as a complication of persistent AOM and is defined as otorrhea through a perforated tympanic membrane for more than 6 weeks.

AOM is an inflammatory condition caused by the presence of microorganisms and often purulent fluid in the middle ear.

AOM is also characterised by a quick onset of otalgia and eardrum erythema. In children otalgia is often accompanied by fever. The disease usually has a self-limiting course, resolving within 8–10 days.

J. Rebol, *Otoscopy Findings*, https://doi.org/10.1007/978-3-031-03979-9_6

6.2   Risk Factors

Known factors for otitis media are as follows:

- gender (more common in male children);
- many children in the family;
- attending in nursery school;
- familiar anamnesis of otitis media;
- use of baby bottle;
- smoking in the home;
- lack of pneumococcal vaccination.

Familial loading is defined by poor immunologic response, anomalies in the middle ear, the palate or the Eustachian tube.

Rare causes are Kartagener syndrome and cystic fibrosis. Socioeconomic factors that can increase the risk are overpopulation, poor diet, and poor access to the health system.

Recently variants of fucose transferase FUT2 gene, important in mucin glycosylation, have been associated with otitis media predisposition [2].

Racial factors also affect the frequency of otitis media because of the differences in Eustachian tube anatomy and skull base (e.g. OM is more common in Native Americans). Food and inhalant allergies and gastroesophageal reflux might also contribute to the development of otitis media, but their precise role has yet to be confirmed.

6.3   Pathogenesis of AOM

Eustachian tube dysfunction, its shorter length, and a more horizontal position of the tube in children compared to adults, contribute to the development secretory otitis. During viral infections of the upper respiratory tract, mucus production in the nasopharynx increases. The mucociliary transport, which prevents the adherence and growth of bacteria, is damaged in viral rhinitis, creating inflammation in the area. Microorganisms in the nasopharynx reflux into the middle ear when the Eustachian tube temporarily relaxes. After bacteria colonise and adhere to the middle ear mucosa, AOM develops.

Bacteria that most commonly cause AOM are *Streptococcus pneumoniae* (12%), nontypable *Haemophilus influenzae* (56%), and *Moraxella catarrhalis* (22%). The incidence of *Streptococcus pneumoniae* related infections has decreased significantly since the implementation of conjugate vaccines. Before the use of vaccines, the percentage of *S. pneumoniae* was much higher—35%. Now the nontypable *Haemophilus influenzae* strains are the ones most commonly isolated. The *Haemophilus influenza* vaccine, part of standard vaccination in children which should prevent pneumonia and meningitis, contains serotype B, which is not a prevalent serotype causing AOM [3]. The vaccine against the Haemophilus and

Moraxella are also being developed. Already by 1995, 25% of Streptococci were resistant to penicillin and a high percentage of Haemophilus and Moraxella were producing beta-lactamase. In children with recurrent AOM, large bacterial colonisation was found at adenotomy. Widespread use of antibiotics for AOM also increases the nasopharyngeal carriage of resistant organisms, which in turn facilitates their spread to other individuals. Antibiotic use promotes more resistance, which in turn promotes more failure and more antibiotic use [4]. Loss of the immunologic function of adenoids and bacterial colonisation of the nasopharynx are important factors in the development of AOM.

Acute middle ear infection with *Haemophilus* species induces a high increase in mucosal secretory capacity, lasting for at least months after the acute incident. *S. pneumoniae* induces the most marked change of bone tissue structures with final osteogenesis. *M. catarrhalis* induces mild changes in the middle ear [5].

Observing children with AOM who are likely to improve without antimicrobial therapy reduces common adverse effects of antibiotics such as diarrhoea and diaper dermatitis.

Clinical diagnosis of AOM is difficult because symptoms of the upper respiratory tract infection may mask those of AOM. Systemic signs that are connected to AOM are fever, otalgia, otorrhea, irritability, and conductive hearing loss. The eardrum is bulged, red, middle ear landmarks are obscured by opaque effusion (Figs. 6.1, 6.2, 6.3, 6.4, and 6.5) [6]. The vascularity of the eardrum is pronounced. If the drum perforates, pus pools in the EAC and otalgia stops immediately. Sometimes the perforation is small and can only be seen after the pus is aspirated and cleaned from the EAC.

Diagnosis is based on otoscopy and functional testing of the eardrum (pneumatic otoscopy and tympanometry). Examination of the child requires experience,

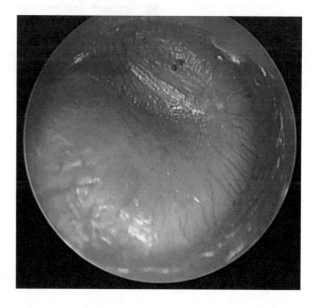

Fig. 6.1 Right ear. The eardrum is slightly bulged and opaque with increased vascularisation at the level of the annulus. The entire middle ear is filled with pus. No middle ear landmarks can be identified

Fig. 6.2 Left ear. The
eardrum is red, swollen,
with a thin layer of pus on
the surface. In the
posterosuperior quadrant a
bulla filled with pus, close
to the perforation, can be
seen. The skin of the EAC
is also red and swollen

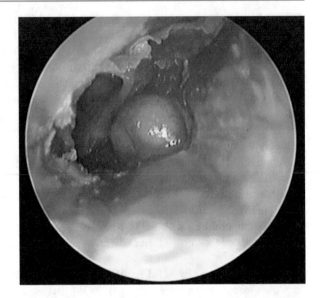

Fig. 6.3 Left ear. The
eardrum is red and
swollen. A bulla occupies
almost the entire eardrum,
the surface epithelium is
cracked. Haemorrhagic
content will most likely be
found inside of the bulla

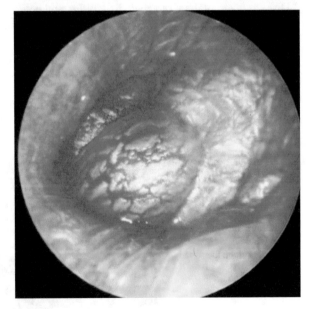

instrument for removal of cerumen from the EAC, and good cooperation of the
health care professional with the parents.

The best tool to differentiate AOM from SOM is pneumatic otoscopy. Reduced
mobility of the eardrum to negative pressure during pneumatic otoscopy is pathog-
nomonic for SOM. Tympanometry may also help to obtain the diagnosis.
Tympanogram type B with a flat curve indicates reduced mobility of the eardrum
due to fluid inside the middle ear. Tympanometry with otoscopy increases the

Fig. 6.4 Left ear. Another case of an opaque eardrum, bulged in the posterior part. The upper part of the eardrum is swollen and red

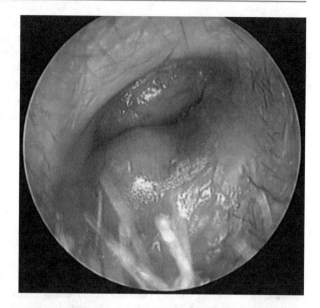

Fig. 6.5 Left ear. The eardrum is very thick and inflamed. In the posterior part polypoid mucosa is protruding through the perforation and pus is oozing from the perforation. Inflammatory changes can also be seen in the mastoid

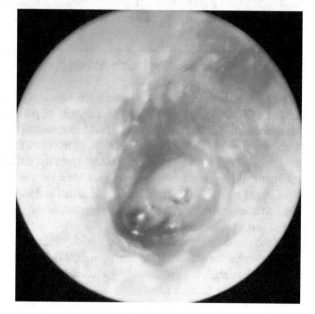

sensitivity and specificity of AOM diagnosis to about 90%. Audiometry shows conductive hearing loss between 20 and 40 dB but is not important for initial diagnosis of AOM. Anamnesis should contain questions about risk factors.

The primary decision is whether observation without antibiotics (watchful waiting) is appropriate for the child. In general antibiotics should be prescribed to children with AOM younger than 6 months, children with severe symptoms (moderate or severe otalgia, otalgia for more than 48 h, or fever above 39 °C) with bilateral or unilateral disease. Antibiotics should also be given to the children younger than 24 months with bilateral disease and to older children with no improvement within 48–72 h after onset of the symptoms [2]. If antibiotic treatment is decided and the last episode of AOM was over 30 days previously, and if the child does not have purulent conjunctivitis caused by beta-lactam resistant *H. influenzae*, amoxicillin dosed at 90 mg/kg per day divided into two doses, should be given. If fewer than 30 days have passed since the last infection or there is concomitant purulent conjunctivitis, amoxicillin plus clavulanate should be used. In case of allergy against penicillin macrolides can be administered.

The goal of antibiotic treatment of AOM is to sterilise the middle ear fluid. Antibiotics need to reach concentrations in the middle ear fluid that are above the minimal inhibitory concentration of the pathogens and remain above this concentration throughout the therapy. In children younger than two, the length of treatment should be 10 days, 7 days for children between the ages of 2 and 5, and 5–7 days for children aged 6 and above [7].

In the future transtympanic drug delivery in children, without the need for systemic antibiotics and surgery could radically change the current treatment paradigm of children with AOM. Higher doses of antibiotics could be delivered topically into the middle ear without systemic effects [8].

6.4   Recurrent Acute Otitis Media

Recurrent AOM is defined as at least three episodes of AOM in 6 months or four episodes of AOM in 12 months. In the majority of patients AOM heals without any complications, but in 10–20% of patients it can lead to the chronic otitis. In patients with recurrent AOM, the risk of developing the chronic disease is higher. The first step should be the removal of risk factors from the child's environment. Persistent inflammation in the middle ear can cause toxic damage to the inner ear—ototoxicity. Longer periods of hearing loss could affect language development. In developing countries, otitis media still represents one of the major causes of hearing loss, which can be prevented.

Prophylactic antibiotic therapy over a long period is not recommended because of growing bacterial resistance. Early surgical intervention is recommended instead of repeated antibiotic treatments. In such cases the insertion of TTs is recommended, in children older than 18 months adenoidectomy can also be performed.

6.5   Complications of AOM

The most common complication of AOM is acute mastoiditis (Figs. 6.6 and 6.7). Incidence could also rise in the future due to of resistant bacteria. Clinically retroauricular swelling can be observed with the skin red and tender. Fever, otalgia, and headache are often present, and there is usually discharge from the EAC. The

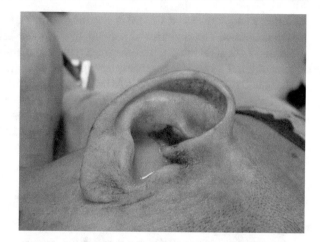

Fig. 6.6 Right ear. The right pinna is protruding due to retroauricular swelling. Pus fills the entrance to the EAC. The patient has otomastoiditis with a subperiosteal abscess

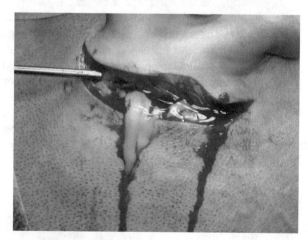

Fig. 6.7 Same patient as in Fig. 6.6. Subperiosteal abscess. Upon incision in the retroauricular region, pus is discharged under pressure. *Streptococcus pneumoniae* was isolated from the swab

condition can lead to subperiosteal abscess, which has to be operated with mastoidectomy and drainage of the abscess. In cases of uncomplicated mastoiditis without subperiosteal abscess, an antibiotic therapy with TT insertion is usually sufficient.

Other complications can include epidural and subdural abscesses, cerebral and cerebellar abscesses, Bezold abscess, labyrinthitis, meningitis, facial paresis, thrombosis of the sigmoid sinus, and the very rare Gradenigo syndrome [3].

6.6 Chronic Suppurative Otitis Media

Chronic suppurative otitis media (CSOM) is defined as chronic otorrhea through a perforated tympanic membrane that is unresponsive to medical treatment [9]. According to WHO, CSOM is defined by 2 weeks of persistent otorrhea. It is estimated that around 20,000 deaths annually are caused by complications of CSOM in children younger than five. CSOM is also the leading cause of hearing loss in developing countries. The majority of patients live in the Western Pacific region, East Asia, and Africa. Otorrhea can come from tympanic membrane perforation or from tympanic tube (TT). CSOM probably develops as a complication of AOM. Organisms isolated in CSOM are different as in AOM, the most common germs are *Pseudomonas aeruginosa*, *Staphylococcus aureus*, *Proteus* spp., *Klebsiella pneumoniae*, diphtheroids, and anaerobes. They are opportunistic pathogens that are difficult to eradicate. Bacteria enter the middle ear from the EAC. Although cerumen contains many antimicrobial substances, its effectiveness against *Pseudomonas* is low. Moisture and heat increase the propensity of these organisms to grow in the EAC and middle ear. They produce toxins which can pass through the round window membrane and cause sensorineural hearing loss. Intracranial complications of CSOM are meningitis, subdural, epidural and brain abscesses, encephalitis, sigmoid sinus thrombosis, and otic hydrocephalus.

In otoscopy we see discharge through the perforated eardrum, which can be purulent, mucoid, serous, or serohemorrhagic. The tympanic membrane is thickened, erythematous. Granulation tissue may surround the perforation and extend to the surface of the eardrum. The middle ear mucosa is oedematous and hyperplastic and may be polypoid (Figs. 6.8, 6.9, 6.10, 6.11, 6.12, 6.13, and 6.14). Treatment for CSOM are topical antibiotic drops either alone or in conjunction with systemic antibiotics. Because of possible ototoxic effect of aminoglycoside drops, the use of topical ciprofloxacin is a safe option. In cases where granulation tissue is present, a biopsy should be performed. If we find no cholesteatoma or granulation tissue, medical therapy based on culture results should be considered. If medical treatment fails, tympanomastoid surgery should be performed.

Fig. 6.8 Left ear. Patient with chronic otorrhea before aspiration. The eardrum is swollen and covered with purulent secretion, partly seen in the posterior half

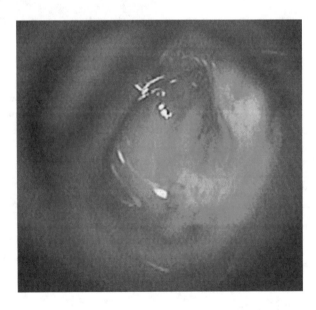

Fig. 6.9 Left ear. Inferior perforation of the eardrum in CSM. The mucosa of the middle ear is swollen and inflamed. In the anterior part of the middle ear an accumulation of mucoid secretion can be seen

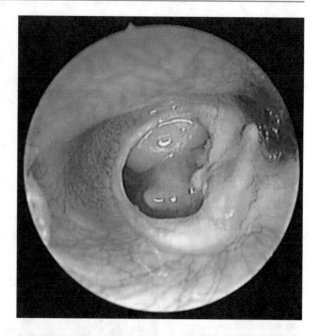

Fig. 6.10 Left ear. Almost the entire lumen of the EAC is obstructed with polypoid tissue surrounded with purulent secretion. The polyp grews from the retraction pocket in the posterior quadrants. Once the polyp is removed, cholesteatoma has to be ruled out

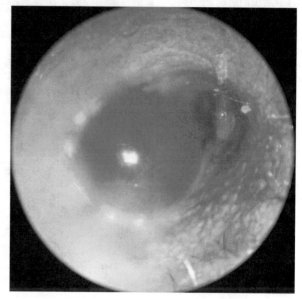

Otorrhea ceases after successful medical therapy and we observe a dry perforation. Because of communication through the perforation with the EAC, otorrhea can reoccur with exacerbation of the middle ear infection. In chronic otitis the perforation of the eardrum usually does not heal spontaneously. Epithelium can also grow from the margins of the perforation under the eardrum, leading to cholesteatoma

Fig. 6.11 Left ear.
Inferior perforation in
patient with CSOM. A
small polyp emerging from
the perforation. The
surface of the eardrum and
the posterior wall of the
EAC are covered with
purulent secretion

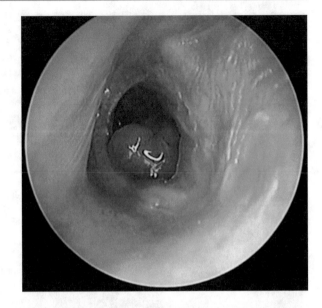

Fig. 6.12 Left ear.
Granulation tissue arising
from the perforation in the
posteroinferior quadrant of
the eardrum

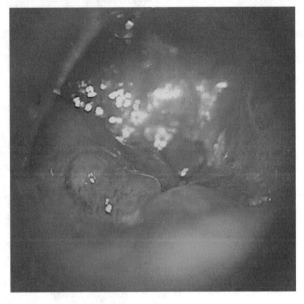

Fig. 6.13 Left ear. Chronic suppurative otitis with purulent secretion in the middle ear, on the eardrum and in the EAC. The perforation is in the anteroinferior quadrant of the eardrum, the rest of the eardrum is red and swollen

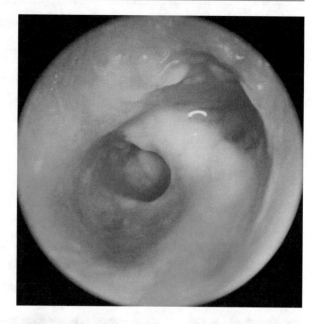

Fig. 6.14 Right ear. Purulent secretion in the EAC with the fungus on the surface of the secretion. The patient has a perforation and permanent secretion from the middle ear

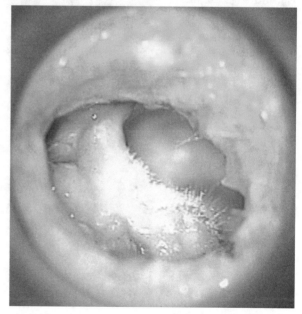

(Fig. 6.15). We distinguish marginal and central perforations. Marginal perforations are located near the annulus and have a greater possibility of growing epithelium under the edges of perforation (Figs. 6.15 and 6.16). With regards to its location, a perforation may exist posterior, inferior, anterior or total (Figs. 6.17, 6.18, 6.19, 6.20, 6.21, 6.22, 6.23, 6.24, 6.25, 6.26, and 6.27).

Fig. 6.15 Right ear.
Marginal perforation in the
posteroinferior quadrant of
the eardrum. The white
epithelium extends on the
inner side of the inferior
part of the eardrum

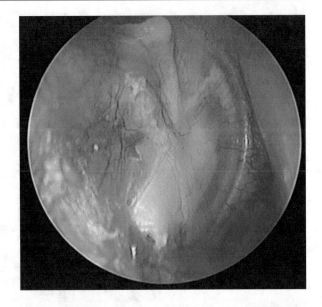

Fig. 6.16 Right ear. The
eardrum is atrophic with
marginal perforation in the
posterosuperior quadrant.
The perforation is dry,
without any ingrowth of
the epithelium

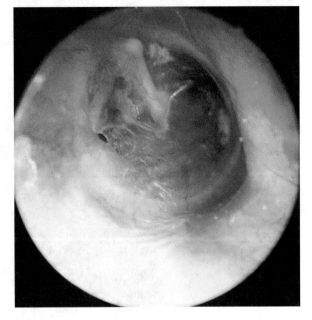

Fig. 6.17 Left ear. Perforation in the posterosuperior quadrant of the eardrum. The stapedial muscle can be seen through the perforation. There is granulation tissue on the edges of the perforation. The patient was treated with local ciprofloxacin drops, which crystalised on the surface of the eardrum

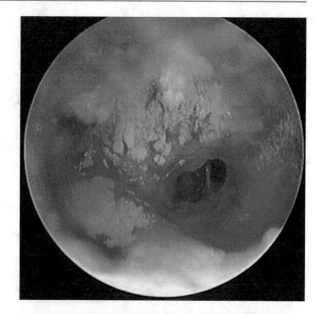

Fig. 6.18 Left ear. The posteriosuperior quadrant of the eardrum is covered with a crust that appeared during spontaneous healing of a perforation

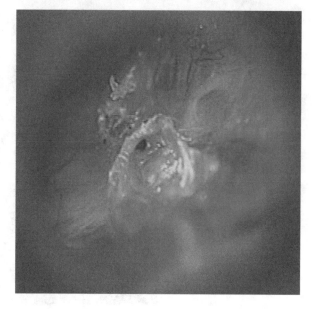

Fig. 6.19 Left ear. Same patient as in the previous figure. The perforation is still present after removal of the crust. Healing was compromised because of the epithelium around the edges of the perforation

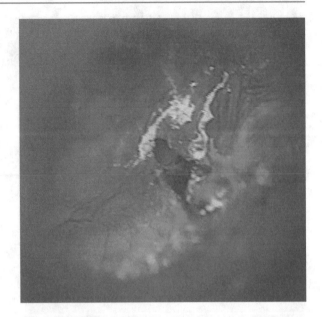

Fig. 6.20 Right ear. Posterior dry perforation of the eardrum. The incudostapedial joint as well as the round window niche in the inferior part can be identified through the perforation

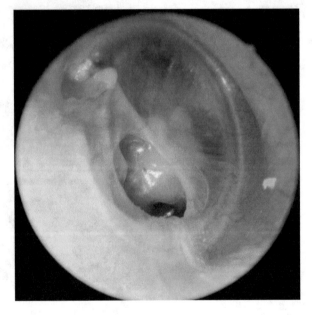

Fig. 6.21 Left ear. Dry posterior perforation of the eardrum. Through the perforation an intact ossicular chain can be seen, as well as the promontory and the round window niche. There is a sclerotic plaque in the anterosuperior quadrant

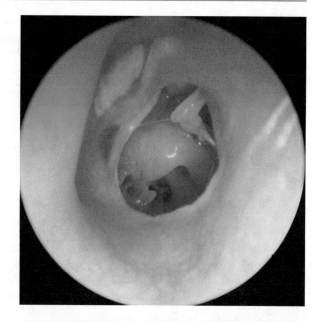

Fig. 6.22 Left ear. Perforation in the posterosuperior quadrant of the eardrum. Through the perforation the pyramidal eminence (PE), the stapedial muscle (SM), the stapes (S), the promontory (P), and the sinus tympani (ST) can be seen

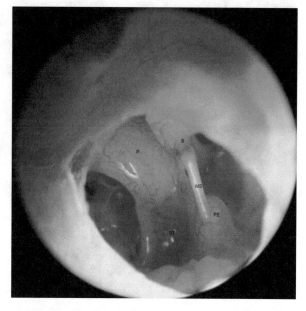

Fig. 6.23 Left ear. Dry
inferior perforation of the
eardrum. A connective
tissue band connects the
umbo with the anterior
margin of the perforation.
Hypotympanic cells can be
seen through the
perforation

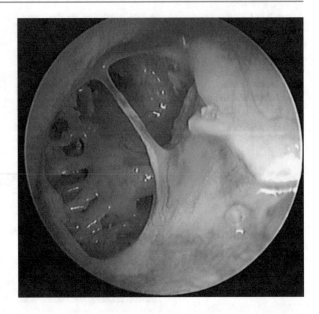

Fig. 6.24 Left ear. The
eardrum is atrophic in the
kidney-shaped area of the
inferior part. Anteriorly
three small perforations
can be observed

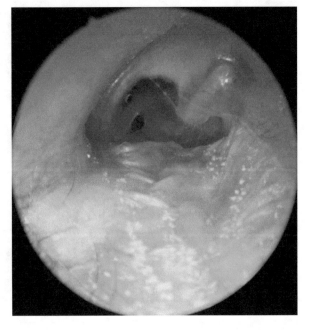

Fig. 6.25 Right ear. The eardrum and the EAC are covered with purulent secretion. There is a small round perforation in the anteroinferior quadrant of the eardrum

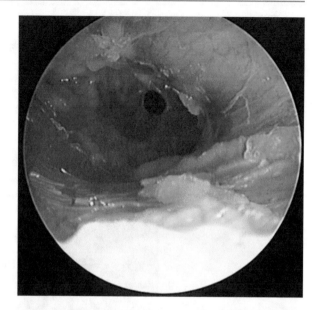

Fig. 6.26 Right ear. Subtotal perforation of the eardrum. The rest of the eardrum is sclerotic and the distal part of malleus handle is also resorbed. The long process of the incus can be identified in the posterosuperior part of the middle ear

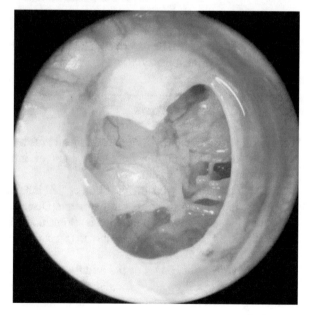

Fig. 6.27 Left ear. Total perforation of the eardrum. The tympanic ostium of the Eustachian tube is in the anterior part of the middle ear. The ossicular chain is missing and the malleus handle is also absent

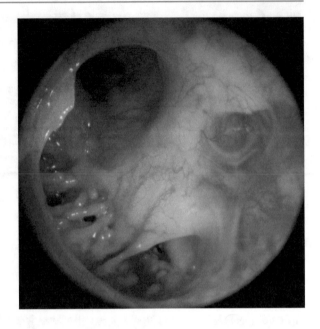

At otoscopy the location of the perforation, its size and if possible, the condition of ossicular chain need to be described. This information is important in planning of the operation—tympanoplasty.

6.7   Tympanosclerosis

Tympanosclerosis is defined as a thickening and fusion of collagenous fibres into a homogeneous mass with the final deposition of intracellular and extracellular calcium and phosphate crystals.

The pathogenesis is probably based on healed inflammation or a particular form of scar tissue following recurrent otitis media. Disease can be limited to the tympanic membrane alone (myringosclerosis) (Figs. 6.28, 6.29, and 6.30) or be present in the middle ear and tympanic membrane (Figs. 6.31 and 6.32). Myringosclerosis can often be observed after TT insertion.

Patients with involvement of the middle ear usually have a large air-bone gap and conductive hearing loss. Ossicular chain fixation often occurs due to deposits around the stapes in the oval niche. If the patient has a perforation, this can first be closed and a stapedectomy can be performed in the second stage. Surgical results differ and are repeatedly unsuccessful. Another option is to offer the patient a hearing aid [10].

Fig. 6.28 Right ear. A large sclerotic plaque on the eardrum. Only a part of malleus handle can be identified. The patient had mild conductive hearing loss

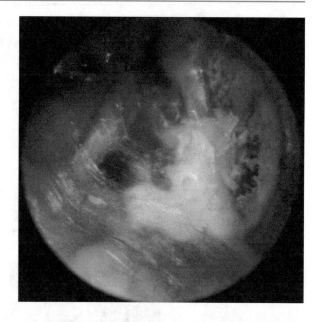

Fig. 6.29 Right ear. Patient had a TT insertion in the past. Kidney-shaped myringosclerosis, only the central part of the eardrum is transparent

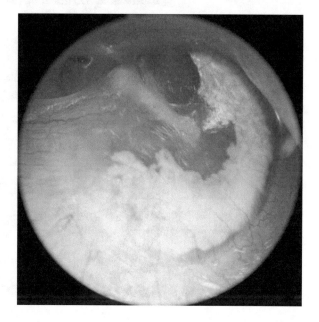

Fig. 6.30 Right ear. The entire eardrum is occupied with a sclerotic plaque

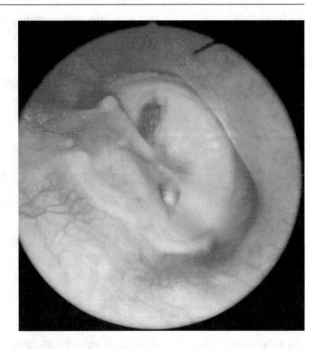

Fig. 6.31 Left ear. The anterior part of the eardrum is almost entirely sclerotic, there is a perforation in the posterior part. Through the perforation white sclerotic masses extend into the oval niche. The patient had a large air-bone gap

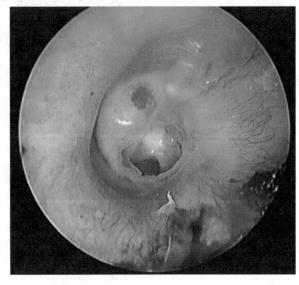

Fig. 6.32 Left ear. Inferior perforation, the rest of the eardrum is white and sclerotic. Sclerotic plaque on the promontory can be seen through the perforation. The patient also has sclerotic changes in the middle ear with ossicular chain fixation

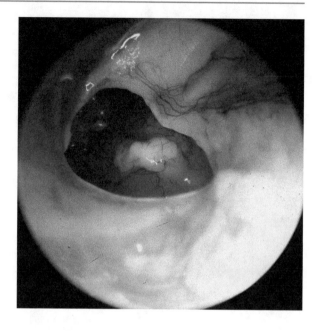

References

1. Raad N, Ghorbani J, Mikaniki N, Haseli S, Karimi-Galougahi M. Otitis media in coronavirus disease 2019: a case series. J Laryngol Otol. 2021;135(1):10–3.
2. Santos-Cortez RLP, Chiong CM, Frank DN, et al. FUT2 variants confer susceptibility to familial otitis media. Am J Hum Genet. 2018;103:679–90.
3. Leichtle A, Hoffmann TK, Wigand MC. Otitis media: definition, pathogenesis, clinical presentation and therapy. Laryngorhinootologie. 2018;97(7):497–508.
4. Dagan R. Treatment of acute otitis media—challenges in the era of antibiotic resistance. Vaccine. 2000;19(Suppl 1):S9–S16.
5. Cayé-Thomasen P, Tos M. Histopathologic differences due to bacterial species in acute otitis media. Int J Pediatr Otorhinolaryngol. 2002;63(2):99–110.
6. Isaacson G. Otoscopic diagnosis of otitis media. Minerva Pediatr. 2016;68(6):470–7.
7. Rosa-Olivares J, Porro A, Rodriguez-Varela M, Riefkohl G, Niroomand-Rad I. Otitis media: to treat, to refer, to do nothing: a review for the practitioner. Pediatr Rev. 2015;36(11):480–6.
8. Shirai N, Preciado D. Otitis media: what is new? Curr Opin Otolaryngol Head Neck Surg. 2019;27(6):495–8.
9. Kenna MA. Treatment of chronic suppurative otitis media. Otolaryngol Clin North Am. 1994;27(3):457–72.
10. Kaur K, Sonkhya N, Bapna AS. Tympanosclerosis revisited. Indian J Otolaryngol Head Neck Surg. 2006;58(2):128–32.

Chronic Otitis Media with Cholesteatoma

7

Cholesteatoma can be defined as the presence of squamous epithelium in the tympanic cavity which normally is lined with respiratory epithelium. It is composed of three layers: the cystic content, the matrix, and the perimatrix. The content of the cyst is fully differentiated keratin squames mixed with purulent and necrotic matter. The matrix consists of stratified squamous epithelium. Perimatrix is the outermost layer; it consists of granulation tissue and inflammatory cells. Cholesteatoma matrix possesses enzymatic activity, which is responsible for osteolysis, leading to ossicular erosions and extension into surrounding structures.

Secondary infection in cholesteatoma is most commonly caused by *Pseudomonas aeruginosa*, *Staphylococcus aureus*, and *Proteus* species.

Most common symptoms are foetid discharge from the EAC, conductive or mixed hearing loss, and sometimes otalgia or headache. Cholesteatoma may cause intracranial complications (meningitis, brain abscess, epidural abscess, septic sinus sigmoideus, and thrombosis of the cavernous sinus). Furthermore it is more aggressive in the paediatric population, where is it more frequently infectious and has a greater recurrence tendency.

The name *cholesteatoma* is misleading (chole = bile, steat = fat, oma = tumour), because it is not composed of fat and is not a tumour. This name appeared in the literature at the beginning of the nineteenth century. The term *keratoma* would be correct and was proposed by Schuknecht in 1974 but was not widely adopted.

The origin of cholesteatoma can be congenital and appears in children or acquired, which can appear in children as well as in adults. Congenital cholesteatoma is typically located in the middle ear under the superior quadrants of the eardrum and may later expand to the entire middle ear. The eardrum in congenital cholesteatoma is intact and patients do not have any history of previous infections. It is assumed that it grows from the epidermal cells that remained in the middle ear during embryonic development (Figs. 7.1 and 7.2).

Acquired cholesteatomas are much more common. They can be further divided into primary acquired and secondary forms. Primary acquired cholesteatoma occurs as a retraction pocket in which desquamated epithelium accumulates and the pocket

J. Rebol, *Otoscopy Findings*, https://doi.org/10.1007/978-3-031-03979-9_7

Fig. 7.1 Right ear. White masses can be seen under the intact eardrum in the posterosuperior quadrant. Surgery confirmed a congenital cholesteatoma

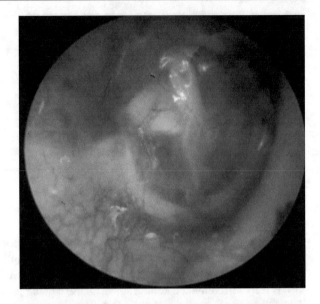

Fig. 7.2 Right ear. Cholesteatoma lesion under an intact eardrum at the level of the posterosuperior quadrant. The 8-year-old patient never reported otalgia or discharge from the ear. Reduced hearing in the right ear was noticed. The cholesteatoma, which also destroyed the long process of the incus and the suprastructure of the stapes, was removed during surgery. A total ossicular replacement prosthesis (TORP) was placed on the stapes footplate

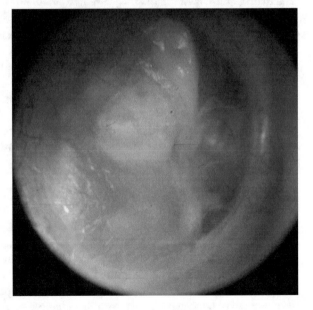

gets inflamed [1]. Secondary cholesteatoma appears after epithelial migration into the middle ear through a perforated eardrum, caused by infection, trauma, or iatrogenically. In 1989 Tos proposed a classification of cholesteatomas into attic (pars flaccida) cholesteatomas, pars tensa cholesteatomas that develop from the retraction of the whole pars tensa of the eardrum, and sinus cholesteatomas that develop from retraction or retraction pockets in the posterosuperior quadrant and extend to the sinus tympani. We now use the EAONO/JOS classification, where the

Fig. 7.3 Right ear. A large attic retraction pocket with a crust. The head of the malleus is partially resorbed. The bottom of the retraction pocket cannot be seen in the posterior and upper parts. There is no sign of cholesteatoma, but such patients need regular follow-ups. In cases of conductive hearing loss, atticotomy, ossiculoplasty, and scutumplasty (reconstruction of the lateral attic wall) can be performed

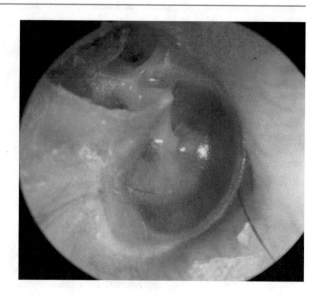

cholesteatomas are divided into congenital, acquired, and unclassifiable forms [2]. Acquired cholesteatomas can be divided into retraction pocket and non-retraction pocket cholesteatomas. Retraction pocket cholesteatomas are further divided into pars flaccida cholesteatomas (Figs. 7.3, 7.4, 7.5, 7.6, 7.7, 7.8, 7.9, 7.10, and 7.11), pars tensa cholesteatomas (Figs. 7.12, 7.13, 7.14, 7.15, 7.16, and 7.17), and a combination of both. Non-retraction cholesteatomas are divided into cholesteatomas following tympanic membrane perforation and iatrogenic or post-traumatic cholesteatomas. In stage I the cholesteatoma is located on the primary site, in stage II it involves more sites, in stage III extracranial complications are present, and in stage IV, the patient has intracranial complications.

Otoscopy is the most important investigation in detecting cholesteatoma. Early detection gives much better chances of removing the cholesteatoma and preserving or improving hearing. Lesions might be overlooked if covered by crusts, debris or granulation tissue. Otoscopy is also important in following up the patients with retraction pockets in which cholesteatoma may potentially occur (Fig. 7.18). The opposite ear should also be examined because the lesion may appear on both sides [3]. Due to osteolytic activity, ossicles are very often eroded (Fig. 7.19).

In planning a surgical approach, a high-resolution CT scan is standard. The images show the extent of the disease and anatomic abnormalities. A scan should always be done in cases of complications (facial paresis, labyrinthine fistula, intracranial complications). Diffusion-weighted magnetic resonance imaging (DW-MRI) is relatively new imaging that also enables the detection of cholesteatoma as well as follow-up in surgically treated patients (non-echo-planar MRI).

Cholesteatoma is treated surgically with the goal of achieving a dry and safe ear, and to restore hearing. Although the treatment is surgical, it is wise to give the patient local antibiotic and corticosteroid drops to reduce inflammation and discharge from the ear prior to surgery. If the infection is extensive, antibiotics may be

Fig. 7.4 Right ear.
Purulent secretion can be
observed in the attic. It is
necessary to aspirate the
secretion carefully
(note—fistula of the lateral
semicircular canal). After
cleaning, keratine masses
with attic perforation
typical for cholesteatoma
were revealed

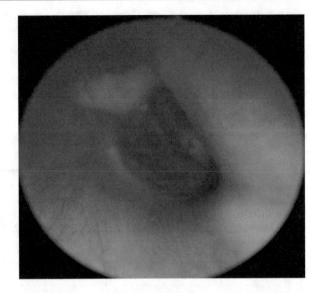

Fig. 7.5 Left ear. A
situation similar to the
previous picture. The
perforation in the attic is
covered with pus, which
has to be cleaned in order
to exclude cholesteatoma.
The pars tensa of the
cholesteatoma is intact

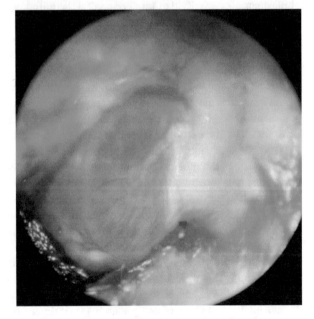

administered systemically. Two types of surgical techniques are performed as
follows.

- Canal wall up (CWU) mastoidectomy: the mastoid cells are removed without
  removing the EAC.
- Canal wall down (CWD) mastoidectomy: the posterior EAC wall is removed and
  a cavity is created that connects the EAC and the mastoid.

Fig. 7.6 Left ear. Small attic perforation with necrotic lesion inside the perforation. Although the perforation is relatively small, the cholesteatoma may extend to the mastoid and the anterior attic

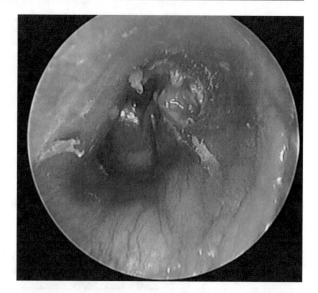

Fig. 7.7 Left ear. Attic perforation with necrotic masses inside of perforation. The eardrum is intact, but is opaque. The head of the malleus and the incus body were resorbed. The cholesteatoma also extended into the middle ear, destroying also the suprastructure of the stapes

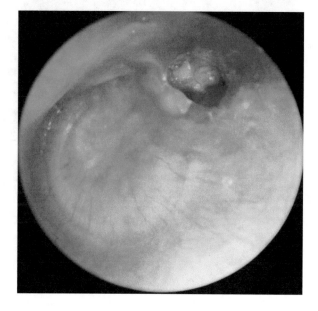

Before the operation we must explain to the patient the goals of surgery. Patients with CWU mastoidectomies require revision surgery ("second look") 12 months after the initial surgery. Children may often require a second or even third operation. Cholesteatoma tends to recur if not completely removed. In operations with an intact canal wall, the chance of improving hearing is much greater than in CWD.

Fig. 7.8 Right ear. Attic cholesteatoma with almost dry keratin squame arising from the attic area. The eardrum is transparent, no cholesteatoma sac can be seen in the middle ear

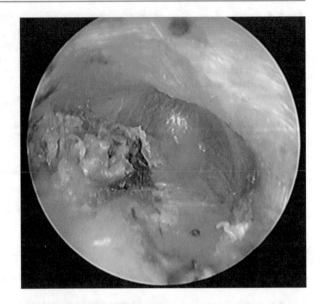

Fig. 7.9 Right ear. The EAC is filled with pus and keratin debris. The eardrum is intact with suppurative secretion coming from the attic. Long lasting purulent secretion with no improvement through therapy is suspicious for cholesteatoma

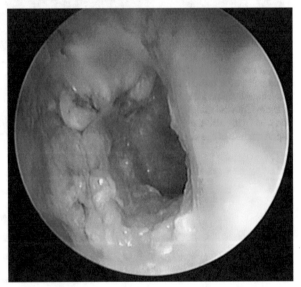

Because of the possibility of recurrence of the disease, patients should be scheduled for follow-ups as long as possible. Patients with CWD mastoidectomy ought to have the cavity cleaned once a year.

Fig. 7.10 Right ear. A brown purulent secretion on the eardrum, a retraction pocket with myringoincudopexy can be seen in the posterior part of the eardrum. There is a perforation in the attic with keratin white masses inside. The presence of keratin in the area where the head of the malleus should be indicates that the ossicles in the attic are eroded

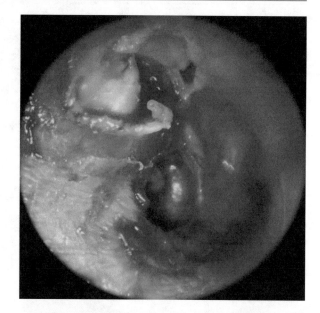

Fig. 7.11 Left ear. There is blood and granulation tissue on the eardrum and a large defect in the attic. The entire cavity is filled with the cholesteatoma, which eroded the lateral attic wall and extends towards the mastoid antrum

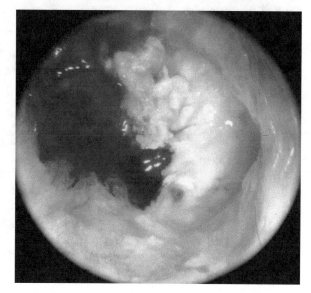

Fig. 7.12 Right ear. Purulent secretion in the EAC. There is granulation tissue in the posterior part of the eardrum. After the removal of the granulation tissue, pars tensa a cholesteatoma with erosion of the long process of the incus and the stapes suprastructure was found

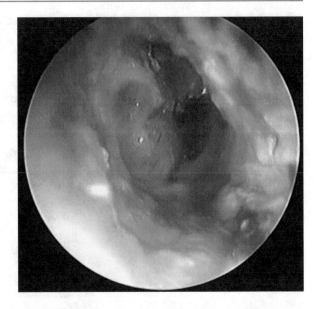

Fig. 7.13 Right ear. Adult patient had many previous episodes of otitis. A worsening of hearing was noticed. A white cholesteatoma sac, bulging above the level of the eardrum in the posterior part can be seen

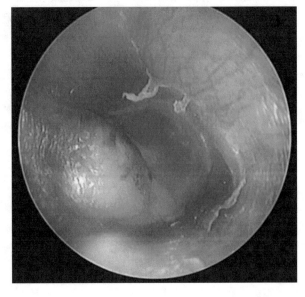

Fig. 7.14 Left ear. Pars tensa cholesteatoma. The posterior perforation in the eardrum is wet. Through the perforation in the upper part a white keratin mass extending towards the attic can be seen. The long process of the incus and the stapes suprastructure are missing. They were eroded by the cholesteatoma

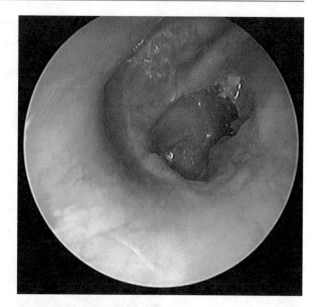

Fig. 7.15 Right ear. Posterior perforation of the eardrum. The mucosa in the middle ear is swollen. Epithelium grew from the edges of the perforation into the middle ear. The rest of the eardrum is white because of the spreading cholesteatoma, which completely fills the anterior part of the middle ear

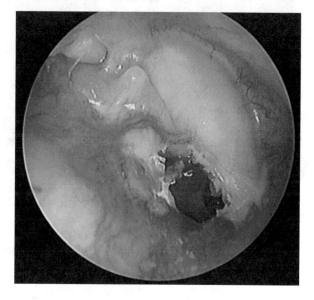

Fig. 7.16 Right ear. Perforation in the posterosuperior quadrant of the eardrum. Squamous epithelium can be seen on the edges and inside the perforation. The cholesteatoma extends to the anterior part of the middle ear. There is a retraction pocket in the inferior part

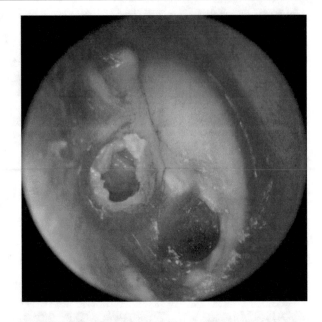

Fig. 7.17 Left ear. A polyp growing from the retraction in the posterosuperior quadrant. After removal of the polyp a cholesteatoma was found in the retraction pocket

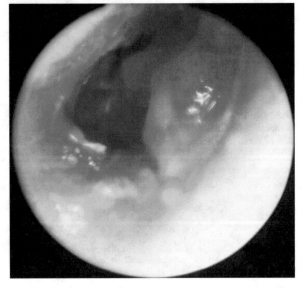

Fig. 7.18 Right ear. White keratin masses in the posterosuperior quadrant of the eardrum have to be cleaned in order to assess the situation. After cleaning the keratin debris, a retraction pocket was visible. The long process of the incus was resorbed. There was flat granulation tissue in the inferior part of the retraction pocket. The bottom of the retraction pocket could not be seen in total

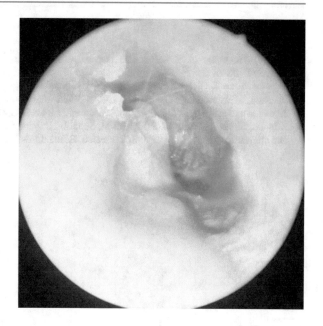

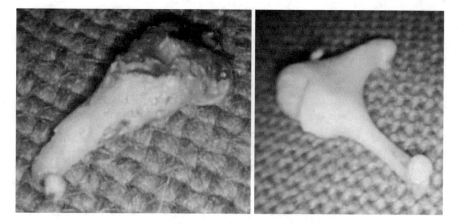

Fig. 7.19 The image on the left shows the incus removed from a patient with attic cholesteatoma, most of the incus body and the short process of the incus are eroded. The image on the right is a normal incus

References

1. Sadé J. Treatment of cholesteatoma and retraction pockets. Eur Arch Otorhinolaryngol. 1993;250:193–9.
2. Yung M, Tono T, Olszewska E, Yamamoto Y, Sudhoff H, Sakagami M, Mulder J, Kojima H, İncesulu A, Trabalzini F, Özgirgin N. EAONO/JOS joint statements on the definitions, classification and staging of middle ear cholesteatoma. J Int Adv Otol. 2017;13(1):1–8.
3. Kuo CL, Shiao AS, Yung M, Sakagami M, Sudhoff H, Wang CH, Hsu CH, Lien CF. Updates and knowledge gaps in cholesteatoma research. Biomed Res Int. 2015;2015:854024.

Temporal Bone Trauma

The temporal bone is injured in up to 70% of head trauma. With improved car safety technologies, the numbers of fractures from car accidents have decreased. Advances in intensive care also enable more patients than previously to survive head trauma. Additional head injuries associated with temporal bone fractures are subdural hematoma, subarachnoid haemorrhage, brain concussion, and tension pneumocephalus [1]. A high-resolution CT (HRCT) with slices of 1 mm is essential for the evaluation of temporal bone fractures.

The temporal bone is very dense and only great forces can cause the injury in this region. Work and traffic-related accidents are also connected to fractures of other bones, prevail. In skull base fractures we have to look at periorbital ecchymosis, mastoid ecchymosis, and hemotympanum (Fig. 8.1). Signs of temporal bone fracture are hearing loss, instability and vertigo, cerebrospinal fluid (CSF) leak, and facial nerve paresis. Less common manifestations include ossicular chain damage, sympathetic sensorineural hearing loss, perilymphatic fistula, cholesteatoma, meningocele, encephalocele, and otogenic meningitis.

Temporal bone fractures were divided into longitudinal and transverse fractions based on observation by Ulrich in 1926 and experiments performed in 1940. Over time patterns of injury have changed and oblique and mixed fractures can also be observed. Longitudinal fractures account for around 80% of temporal bone fractures and are caused by forces that come from lateral side along the petrosquamous suture. Facial nerve paresis is present in 15–20% of longitudinal fractures, we also often observe laceration of the EAC (Figs. 8.2, 8.3, 8.4, and 8.5). Transverse fractures are caused by forces in an anteroposterior direction. Facial nerve injury occurs in the labyrinthine portion and the nerve is frequently transected, while in longitudinal fractures transection of the nerve is rarely seen.

About 70% of patients with temporal bone fracture have ossicular chain injuries, which include dislocation at the incudomallear and incudostapedial joints, and fractures of the malleus and stapes. Patients should undergo an audiometry test 4–6 weeks after the injury. By then any hemotympanum is already resorbed. If the air bone gap at audiometry is greater than 40 dB, the patient probably has an

J. Rebol, *Otoscopy Findings*, https://doi.org/10.1007/978-3-031-03979-9_8

Fig. 8.1 Right ear. Hemotympanum—blood fills the entire middle ear, the tympanic membrane is intact. Patients has conductive hearing loss. Hemotympanum can be an indirect sign of temporal bone fracture

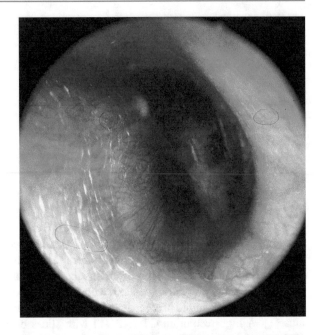

Fig. 8.2 Right ear. After removal of soft tissues, a longitudinal temporal bone fracture can be seen in the posterior wall of the EAC, running from the middle ear in a lateral direction. Posteriorly the lateral part of mastoidectomy was drilled. The fracture line also goes through the mastoid in a retromastoid direction. The patient was operated because of facial paralysis

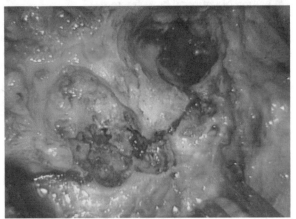

ossicular discontinuity (Figs. 8.6, 8.7, and 8.8). In transverse fractures sensorineural hearing loss is usually present, with little chance of improvement.

Vertigo is the consequence of a fracture through the otic capsule, vestibular concussion or perilymph fistula. Instability usually resolves after 1 year with central adaptation. The disorder is managed with rest, diminished activity, vestibular suppressants, antiemetics and, after time, gradual activation.

CSF leak manifests with a watery discharge from the ear (Fig. 8.9). The discharge can also appear from the nose. CSF leak is managed conservatively with head elevation, bed rest, stool softeners, avoidance of nose blowing. CSF can be collected to determine the presence of beta 2 transferrine or beta trace protein. If the

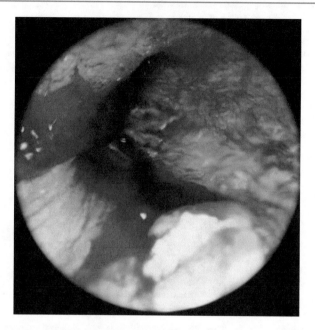

Fig. 8.3 Left ear. Acute temporal bone fracture. The skin of the EAC is swollen, there is blood in the fracture line and the anterior wall of the EAC is also fractured. Only the posterior part of the eardrum can be seen with the perforation in the posteroinferior quadrant. There is blood in the middle ear. The patient had facial nerve paralysis, the facial nerve was injured at the level of the second genu. They also had conductive hearing loss because of the hemotympanum and ossicular chain disruption at the level of incudostapedial joint

Fig. 8.4 Right ear. Patient after the healed longitudinal temporal bone fracture. The fracture line, running from the middle ear in the lateral direction, can still be identified under the intact skin. The patient had a haematoma around the facial nerve in the horizontal part

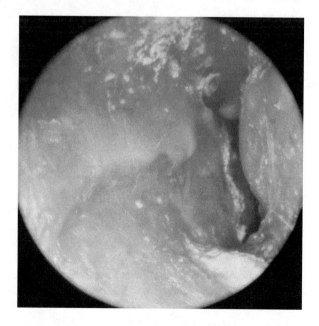

Fig. 8.5   Right ear.
Another example after the
fracture of the temporal
bone. The patient was
injured as a cyclist, also
had other injuries and was
in an artificial coma for
many months. The injured
ear was deaf, with normal
function of the facial nerve

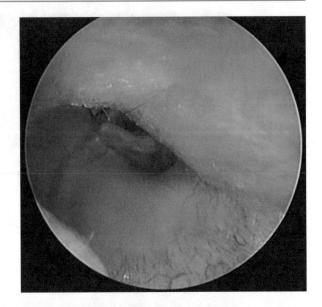

Fig. 8.6   Left ear. After
temporal bone fracture the
patient suffered from
conductive hearing loss. At
surgery a dislocated
incudostapedial joint was
found. The tympanomeatal
flap was raised to look
inside the middle ear. The
lenticular process of the
incus is not completely
covering the head of the
stapes

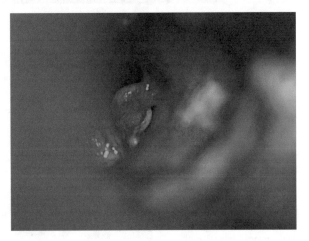

CSF leak persists for more than 2 weeks, it is possible that no spontaneous healing
will occur and surgical therapy will be needed (Fig. 8.10). It is advisable to pre-
scribe antibiotic prophylaxis to prevent the development of meningitis.

In temporal bone fractures, facial nerve function should always be assessed. The
timing of the onset of paresis is important in decision making and in the prognosis
for facial nerve function. It is also important to determine whether the patient has
paresis or facial nerve paralysis. Immediate paralysis indicates a transection of the
nerve, whereas delayed onset paresis usually follows after a haematoma or oedema
of the facial nerve. With immediate paralysis of the facial nerve, surgery is advocated. Patients with delayed onset and incomplete paresis should be treated with

Fig. 8.7 Left ear. The patient is a young man received a head injury while cycling. The temporal bone was fractured and the stapes and incus were separated. The lenticular process of the incus is prominent above the level of the tympanic membrane in the posterosuperior quadrant. The incus was shaped and placed as an interposition graft between the head of stapes and the handle of malleus. The patient's hearing returned to almost normal after the procedure

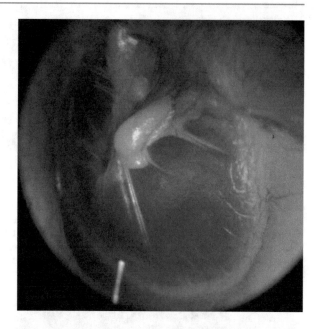

Fig. 8.8 Right ear. After falling from a bunk bed, patient had conductive hearing loss. In surgery we found that both crura of the stapes were fractured. The stapedial defect was overcome with a prosthesis

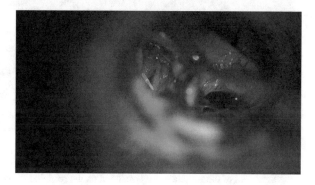

high-dose corticosteroids and investigated with electrophysiologic examinations (electroneuronography and electromyography).

Structures of the temporal bone can also be injured without fracture of the temporal bone [2]. Such injuries can be caused by barotrauma as well as thermal, foreign body, and compressive injuries. Traumatic perforation of the tympanic membrane is commonly seen in accident and emergency departments. It is accompanied by conductive hearing loss that correlates with the size of the perforation (Figs. 8.11 and 8.12) [3]. Traumatic perforation can be caused by blunt trauma (overpressure), penetrating trauma (cotton swab), barotrauma, and blast injuries. Best management is controversial. Spontaneous healing with water precaution occurs in up to 95% of cases. Perforation can be also covered with various materials such as cigarette paper, fat, gelatine film or silk to enhance the healing [4] (Figs. 8.13, 8.14, and 8.15). Healing of the perforation may be delayed, if the water enters the ear, causing otitis media (Fig. 8.16).

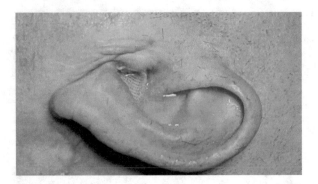

Fig. 8.9 Patient after head injury with fracture of the temporal bone with bone defect and tear of the middle cranial fossa dura. In the cavitas conchae is a collection cerebrospinal fluid (CSF). The patient was admitted to the intensive care unit, where CSF leak did not stop or was even reduced after 10 days of conservative treatment. The dural defect was closed through the transmastoid route. Temporalis muscle facia and artificial dura were used to close the defect

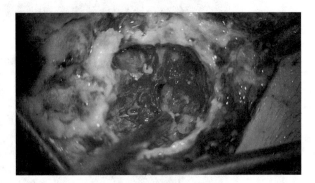

Fig. 8.10 Left ear. The tip of the aspirator is pointing towards an encephalocele with CSF leak after the temporal bone fracture. The patient was injured in a traffic accident during which they were thrust out of the vehicle and resuscitated on the roadside. They spent a long time in intensive care and presented CSF leak behind the intact tympanic membrane. Closure of the CSF leak was advised but the patient refused. Meningitis and encephalitis developed soon after and surgery was performed. After the closure of the defect in the middle fossa dura, the patient's condition improved

Fig. 8.11 Right ear. Triangle shaped traumatic perforation of the tympanic membrane in the anteroinferior quadrant. The perforation is dry, with a small flap at the anterior edge of the perforation

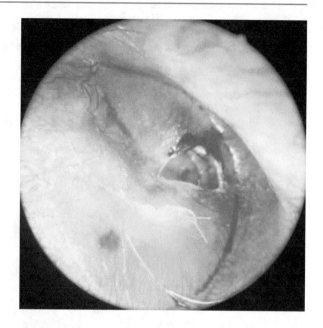

Fig. 8.12 Left ear. Traumatic perforation located in the posterosuperior quadrant of the tympanic membrane. An intact incudostapedial joint is visible through the perforation. There is a flap on the anterior edge of the perforation, adherent to the surface of the tympanic membrane. It can be repositioned to reduce the size of the perforation

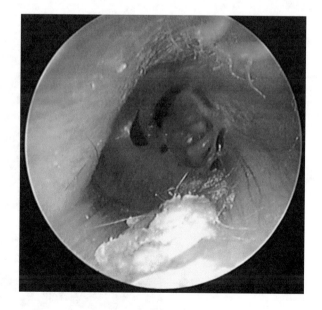

Fig. 8.13 Left ear. Traumatic perforation in the anteroinferior quadrant of the tympanic membrane. The anterior edge of the perforation cannot be seen because of the prominent anterior wall of the EAC

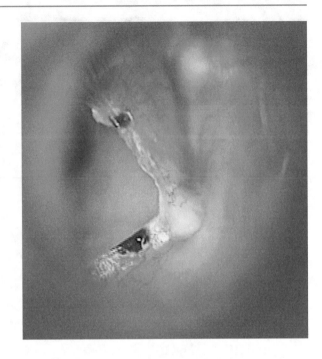

Fig. 8.14 The same patient as shown in Fig. 8.13. With a hooked needle the triangular flap at the anterior edge of the perforation could be mobilised and is covering a large part of the perforation. The chances of spontaneous healing are high

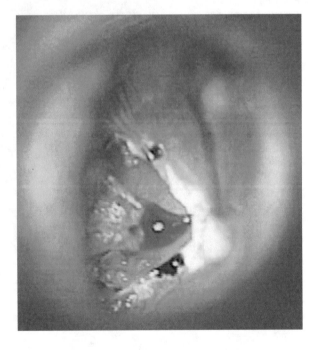

Fig. 8.15 The same patient as shown in Figs. 8.13 and 8.14. A sterile nylon mesh was placed on the repositioned tympanic membrane flap. This will hold it in place until spontaneous healing. The mesh is removed from the tympanic membrane after 6 weeks. By then the perforation usually already heals

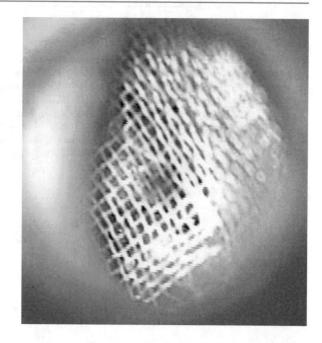

Fig. 8.16 Left ear. Central traumatic perforation. The tympanic membrane is red and wet on the surface. There is a small flap on the posterior edge. The patient jumped into water, which entered the middle ear, causing acute otitis. They needed antibiotic therapy

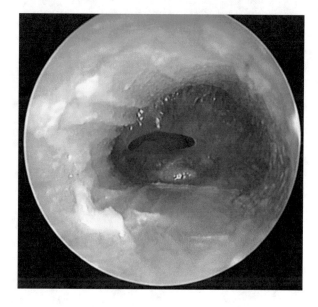

References

1. Johnson F, Semaan MT, Magerian CA. Temporal bone fracture: evaluation and management in the modern era. Otolaryngol Clin North Am. 2008;41:597–618.
2. Huang MY, Lambert PR. Temporal bone trauma. In: Hughes GB, Pensak ML, editors. Clinical otology. 3rd ed. New York: Thieme; 2007. p. 273–88.
3. Sagiv D, Migirov L, Glikson E, Mansour J, Yousovich R, Wolf M, Shapira Y. Traumatic perforation of the tympanic membrane: a review of 80 cases. J Emerg Med. 2018;54(2):186–90.
4. Cayir S, Mutlu H. Traumatic tympanic membrane perforation in children in the emergency department: comparison of spontaneous closure and the paper patch. Cureus. 2020;12(4):e7697.

Paraganglioma

9

The most common tumours of the temporal bone are vestibular schwannomas. A vestibular schwannoma is located in the internal acoustic meatus and cannot be discovered at otoscopy. Asymmetric hearing loss, tinnitus, and vestibular dysfunction are the symptoms that lead us towards further investigations.

Paragangliomas are the most common tumours of the middle ear. Tumours that arise from the Jacobson's nerve are called tympanic paragangliomas, ones that arise from the jugular bulb are called jugular paragangliomas. Paragangliomas are neuroendocrine tumours arising from extra-adrenal paraganglia of the autonomic nervous system [1, 2].

Jugular paragangliomas are rare, slow-growing tumours arising from paraganglia cells in the adventitia of jugular bulb. Because of their low prevalence, slow growth, and hidden location at physical examination, the disease is usually quite advanced at diagnosis, with symptoms lasting years [3, 4].

In the literature paragangliomas are traditionally named glomus tumours, due to the prevalent opinion that chief (neurosecretion) cells of paragangliomas originate from vessel wall pericytes, as is true with actual glomus tumours found in skin. However, paraganglia cells have a neuroectodermal origin and bear no connection to these arteriovenous malformations [5, 6].

Nonchromaffin paraganglia are mostly microscopic bodies, consisting of lobules of epithelioid cells nested in a richly vascularised stroma. They are located along the cranial nerves containing autonomous fibres, e.g. the glossopharyngeal nerve and the vagal nerve. They are capable of producing and storing biogenic monoamines (catecholamines and serotonin). The best-studied are the functions of paraganglia associated with the carotid and aortic bodies, which are known to serve as chemoreceptors.

Other nonchromaffin paraganglia are structurally identical, but their chemoreceptor function has never been proven. The anatomic placement of temporal bone paraganglia is inconsistent but is always related to the course the Jacobson nerve (n. tympanicus) and the Arnold's nerve (the auricular branch of the vagus nerve).

J. Rebol, *Otoscopy Findings*, https://doi.org/10.1007/978-3-031-03979-9_9

The incidence of jugulotympanic (temporal) paraganglioma is approximately 1:1.3 million [7]. They are the second commonest tumours of the temporal bone and are 4–6 times more frequent in women than men. In women they most often appear sporadically between the age of 40 and 60. In men, hereditary forms are relatively more common and appear at younger age.

Multicentric paragangliomas appear in 10–20% of sporadic and up to 80% of hereditary cases. Mostly they are benign with only around 2–4% being malignant [8].

Hearing loss and pulsatile tinnitus are the most frequent symptoms at presentation. Pain and vertigo are somewhat less common. When the tympanic membrane is injured by the tumour, ear discharge or haemorrhage can be seen. Signs of compression of cranial nerves VII, IX, X, XI, and XII are often seen as facial palsy, dysphagia, hoarseness, shoulder elevation palsy, and tongue hemiparesis, respectfully. At otoscopy the tympanic membrane can be intact with a reddish tumour behind it or red polypoid tissue in ear canal (Figs. 9.1, 9.2, 9.3, 9.4, 9.5, and 9.6). When the tumour grows intracranially, signs of high intracranial pressure can join the clinical presentation.

Besides thorough clinical examination, contrast enhanced computed tomography and/or magnetic resonance imaging is essential. A diffuse-type infiltrative growth pattern with bone erosion and high contrast uptake can be seen, which differentiates it from a meningioma or schwannoma. The latter two also rarely invade the middle ear. A four-vessel angiography is needed at preoperative planning to show the vascular anatomy of the tumour, the possibility of preoperative embolisation, and intracranial circulation. The Fisch classification of temporal paragangliomas is most often used for grading tumour size [9].

Treatment of jugular paragangliomas is demanding and requires a team approach. Surgical treatment with the goal of not creating further cranial nerve deficits is

Fig. 9.1 Left ear. There is red tumour tissue in the anteroinferior quadrant, touching the tympanic membrane. The patient had pulsatile tinnitus and conductive hearing loss. The tumour was removed using the transcanal approach. It is a tympanic paraganglioma because it grew from the promontory

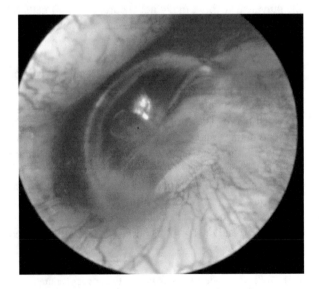

Fig. 9.2 Right ear. A red tumour can be seen through the transparent tympanic membrane. It has a typical "rising sun" appearance that we commonly observe in jugular paragangliomas. Under magnification the pulsation of the tumour can be observed

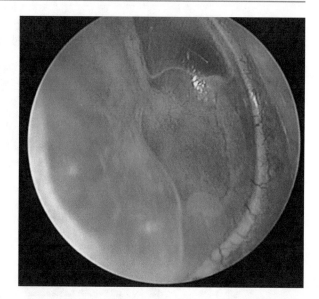

Fig. 9.3 Right ear. Another patient with a jugular paraganglioma tumour. The tumour is present only in the hypotympanic region of the middle ear. Patterns of growth of these tumours are different. Although the tumour appears to be small, it grew along the carotid canals and was pressing on the lower cranial nerves. The patient had vagus, glossopharyngeal, and hypoglossal nerve paralysis

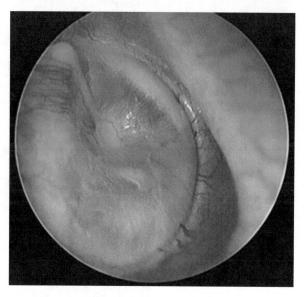

mostly the therapy of choice. Preoperatively, a CT angiography is done to demonstrate intracranial arterial and venous circulation and tumour embolisation options. Embolisation is usually performed via an arterial approach by way of superselective catheterisation and embolisation of the supplying arteries. The Fisch type-A infratemporal fossa approach is most frequently utilised to access the tumour. This is done with a retroauricular cut and radical mastoidectomy. The facial nerve is mobilised from its bony canal distally to the geniculate ganglion and transposed anteriorly. The sigmoid sinus is then ligated and the remaining part of the mastoid and

Fig. 9.4 Left ear. Almost
the entire tympanic
membrane is bulged due to
the red pulsating tumour. A
CT scan showed it was a
tympanic paraganglioma
with extension into the
bony part of the Eustachian
tube and into the attic. The
patient had no lower
cranial nerve deficits

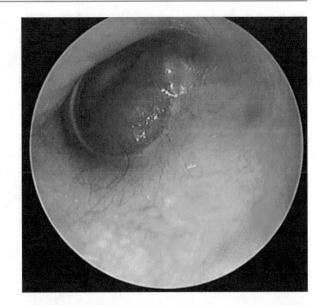

Fig. 9.5 Left ear. Jugular
paraganglioma, that was
growing from the jugular
bulb, extending into the
mastoid and the middle
ear. In otoscopy the
tympanic membrane
appears bulged in the
posterior part, which was
pulsating. The patient had
no nerve deficits and was
operated through the
infratemporal fossa
approach with anterior
rerouting of the facial
nerve

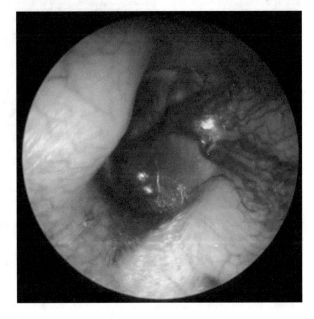

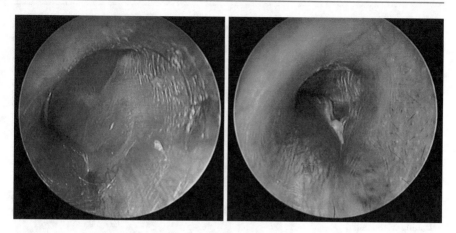

Fig. 9.6 Left ear. The patient visited the doctor because of pulsatile tinnitus and conductive hearing loss. On the left figure a vascularised tumour in the inferior part of the middle ear can be seen. It has a typical "rising sun" appearance. The tumour can also be seen in front of the eardrum, where the ear canal is elevated. A CT scan with contrast showed that the patient has a jugular paraganglioma. They had no cranial nerve palsies and chose observation of the tumour rather than immediate surgical treatment. After 4 years the tumour had grown considerably although the growth rate of this kind of tumours is very slow. The tumour in the EAC now covers the inferior part of the tympanic membrane. The rest of the tympanic membrane is red due to the tumour spreading into the entire middle ear

styloid process removed to fully expose jugular fossa. The tumour can then be extirpated along with the lateral wall of sigmoid sinus. The internal jugular vein is ligated (Fig. 9.7). The tissue gap is then filled with abdominal fat and additional support can be provided by inferior rotation of the temporal muscle. A secondary treatment option is (stereotactic) radiation, usually considered in inoperable, recurrent or residual tumours (Fig. 9.8).

Surgical procedure cannot restore any nerve palsies seen preoperatively. One of the palsies with the most bothersome effects in everyday life is vagal nerve paralysis that causes dysphonia and, most notably, dysphagia with the risk of aspiration. Other tumours of the middle ear are very rare (Fig. 9.9).

In tympanic paragangliomas surgical therapy is the treatment of choice. If they are limited to the tympanic cavity only, they can be removed using transcanal approach.

Fig. 9.7 The postoperative specimen of the jugular vein bulb of the patient from the previous figure. In the upper part it transected the sigmoid sinus, in the lower part the internal jugular vein. The tumour was removed from the mastoid and the middle ear. The bulb is protuberant due to tumour tissue within the vessel. The patient had transient facial nerve paresis following anterior rerouting of the facial nerve during the operation. The lower cranial nerves remained intact without any paresis. The patient's pulsatile tinnitus also disappeared

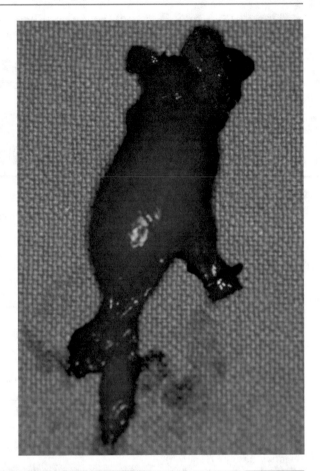

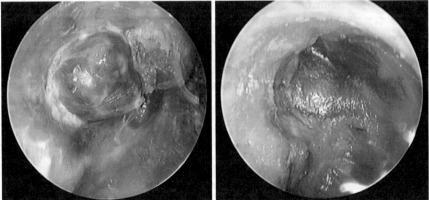

Fig. 9.8 Left ear. The patient was referred from another institution after an attempted removal of the paraganglioma simply through canal wall down mastoidectomy (CWD). On the left, the tumour can be seen in the cavity. With a CT scan with contrast an aplastic transverse venous sinus was identified on the contralateral side. This meant that surgical removal of the tumour was not possible and the patient proceeded with stereotactic radiotherapy. The image on the right shows a significant reduction of the tumour after the radiotherapy

Fig. 9.9 Left ear. Adenoma of the middle ear. The patient visited the doctor due to conductive hearing loss. The eardrum is intact, underneath it is a yellow mass which occupies most of the middle ear. Diagnosis was made by tympanoscopy and biopsy of the tumour. Treatment is surgical

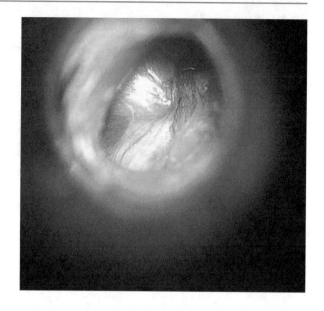

References

1. Pellitteri P. Paragangliomas of the head and neck. Oral Oncol. 2004;40(6):563–75.
2. Capatina C, Ntali G, Karavitaki N, Grossman AB. The management of head-and-neck paragangliomas. Endocr Relat Cancer. 2013;20(5):R291–305.
3. Carlson ML, Sweeney AD, Wanna GB, Netterville JL, Haynes DS. Natural history of glomus jugulare: a review of 16 tumors managed with primary observation. Otolaryngol Head Neck Surg. 2015;152(1):98–105.
4. Sokabe A, Mizooka M, Sakemi R, Kobayashi T, Kishikawa N, Yokobayashi K, et al. Systemic inflammatory syndrome associated with a case of jugular paraganglioma. Intern Med. 2016;55(15):2105–8.
5. Myssiorek D. Head and neck paragangliomas: an overview. Otolaryngol Clin North Am. 2001;34(5):829–36.
6. Forbes JA, Brock AA, Ghiassi M, Thompson RC, Haynes DS, Tsai BS. Jugulotympanic paragangliomas: 75 years of evolution in understanding. Neurosurg Focus. 2012;33(2):E13.
7. Woolen S, Gemmete JJ. Paragangliomas of the head and neck. Neuroimaging Clin N Am. 2016;26(2):259–78.
8. Gulya AJ. The glomus tumor and its biology. Laryngoscope. 1993;103(11 Pt 2 Suppl 60):7–15.
9. Wanna GB, Sweeney AD, Haynes DS, Carlson ML. Contemporary management of jugular paragangliomas. Otolaryngol Clin North Am. 2015;48(2):331–41.

Cochlear Implants

10

Otology can nowadays offer a solution almost for all kinds of hearing loss. Important progress in hearing loss restoration has been made with cochlear implantation. It began over 30 years ago with the development of the multichannel cochlear implant. Patients with severe to profound hearing loss are candidates for the operation. When the electrode is inserted into the cochlea, the cochlear nerve is stimulated and the stimulus is propagated in the central nervous system.

Developments in programming strategies, device design, and minimal traumatic surgical techniques have contributed to safety and efficacy of cochlear implant (CI) surgery. Cochlear implantation is one of the highest-ranked medical interventions with regard to cost-effectiveness, especially in children. The rate of assignment to mainstream schooling within 5 years of cochlear implantation has increased to 75% of operated children. Adults with CI achieve hearing thresholds between 25 and 30 dB and about 60% are able to use the telephone for everyday communication and social interaction. The device also enables the patient to converse without lip reading (especially important during the pandemic when people wear face masks) and reduces depression symptoms that are common in people with hearing loss.

In children the indications for CI are bilateral sensorineural hearing loss which is severe (71–90 dB) to profound (over 90 dB). Children with this degree of hearing loss have no or minimum benefit from a 3–6 months hearing aid trial period. Hearing loss can be prelingual, perilingual or post-lingual. Imaging tests should show the presence of the cochlear nerve and the absence of alterations in the auditory pathway. Better results are related to early intervention. Children can be operated on even at an age younger than 12 months. The operation can be performed once the child has gained 7 kg. A bilateral implantation can be done simultaneously or sequentially [1]. Whenever possible, it is better to perform a simultaneous bilateral cochlear implantation. If this is not feasible, the time between implantations should be as short as possible [2].

In adults the indication is also severe (71–90 dB) to profound (over 90 dB) bilateral sensorineural hearing loss. Hearing loss can be prelingual or post-lingual. Candidates for implantation have no or minimum benefit from hearing aid and

J. Rebol, *Otoscopy Findings*, https://doi.org/10.1007/978-3-031-03979-9_10

understand less than 40% of words at 65 dB SPL after a trial period of 3–6 months. Prior psychological evaluation is also recommended.

In asymmetrical hearing loss (severe to profound hearing loss in one ear and moderate to severe on the other), cochlear implantation would be done on the worst-affected ear and a hearing aid can be used on the other ear. Such treatment is called bimodal stimulation.

Imaging tests should also be performed on the CI candidate to determine the presence of the cochlear nerve and whether the cochlea is patent (Figs. 10.1 and 10.2). Imaging should help exclude the presence of any primary and secondary bony lesions that affect the cochlea, and should evaluate the appearance of the internal auditory canal, pneumatisation of the mastoid and the middle ear, the size of the vestibular aqueduct, and any cochlea-vestibular malformations.

Fig. 10.1 A 3D MRI reconstruction of the inner ear done before cochlear implantation. The cochlea is patent and has two and a half turns. The semicircular canals can also be seen

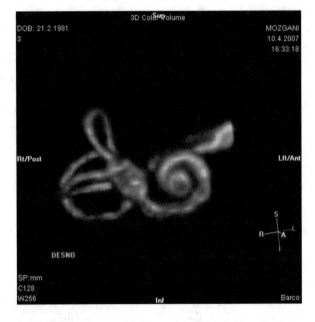

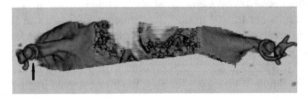

Fig. 10.2 A bilateral 3D MRI reconstruction of the inner ear. The patient suffered from meningitis many years previously and had been deaf in the right ear ever since. On the right side the basal turn of the cochlea cannot be shown due to ossification in that part of the cochlea (arrow). Compare to the other side which has a normal anatomy. During cochlear implantation the electrode was inserted through the middle turn of the cochlea

Fig. 10.3 The inner part of a cochlear implant with the receiver and the electrode, which is pre-shaped and bends around the modiolus after insertion into the cochlea

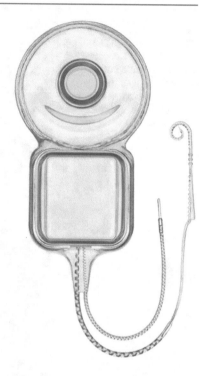

After an audiological and radiographic evaluation, the aetiology of hearing loss should also be determined. The duration of hearing loss is also a valuable information.

The CI consists of external and internal components. The external components include a microphone, battery, speech processor, external magnet, and a transmitter antenna. The internal part includes an internal magnet, antenna, receiver-stimulator, and an electrode array (Figs. 10.3 and 10.4).

The operation is carried out under general anaesthesia and without muscle relaxation to enable facial nerve monitoring during the operation. A mastoidectomy with posterior tympanotomy is performed to gain access to the cochlea (Fig. 10.5). The electrode can be introduced through the round window (Figs. 10.6 and 10.7) or by cochleostomy (creating an opening in the basal turn of the cochlea). The electrode should be inserted to the scala tympani in the cochlea, where the electrode is close to the auditory nerve. Such insertion improves speech understanding after the surgery. In majority of cases the well for the implant body is drilled out in the outer cortex of the skull. In some cases, a tight subperiosteal pocket can be created [3, 4]. The position of the electrode inside of the cochlea can be controlled during or after the surgery (Fig. 10.8).

Two to four weeks after surgery, when the surgical incision has healed, the device is activated. Device programming continues over time and the sound quality in patients improves during the first 6 months or even longer. Better results are achieved in patients with lower age at implantation, shorter length of deafness, previous

Fig. 10.4 Patient with a "behind the ear" (BTE) external part of a cochlear implant consisting of a microphone, speech processor and a transmitter, attached to the inner part with a magnet

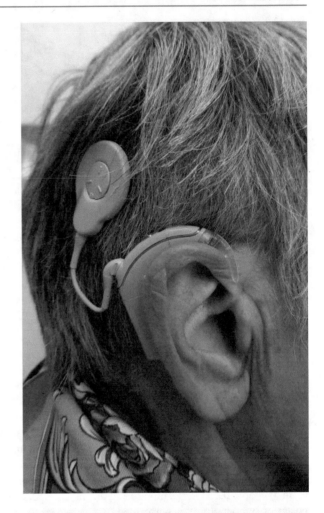

Fig. 10.5 Left ear. The first stage of cochlear implantation. A mastoidectomy, atticotomy, and posterior tympanotomy are carried out by drilling. The round window can be identified through the posterior tympanotomy

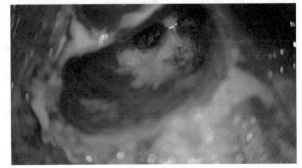

Fig. 10.6 The same patient as shown in Fig. 10.5. The round window membrane is incised in preparation for inserting the electrode

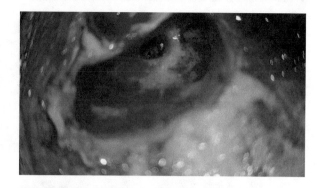

Fig. 10.7 The same patient as shown in Figs. 10.5 and 10.6. The body of the implant is positioned inside the well drilled into the temporal bone. The reference electrode is positioned under the temporalis muscle and the electrode is inserted into the cochlea through the round window

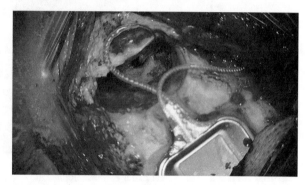

experience with sound, and good access to rehabilitation and therapy services. The motivation of the patient and the parents also plays an important role.

In the past MRI was contraindicated or conditionally indicated (1.5 T magnetic field) in patients with CI. The magnetic field can induce malfunctioning in the device or injure the patient due to heating, migration of the magnet, or even torqueing of the device. Newer generations of cochlear implants enable the exposure to the magnetic field up to 3.0 T with a head bandage [4].

Complications in cochlear implantation are rare. They can be divided into early and late complications. The main early complications are infection, facial paresis, eardrum perforation, facial nerve stimulation, otalgia, vertigo, tinnitus, and loss of taste. Late complications are skin flap problems, cholesteatoma, migration of the electrode, and device failure [5]. Biofilm formation can occur even years after a successful implantation and can lead to explanation of the device [6]. A swelling in the region of the implant body indicates such a complication (Figs. 10.9 and 10.10).

Fig. 10.8 Transorbital
projection in a child after
bilateral cochlear
implantation with slim
straight electrodes

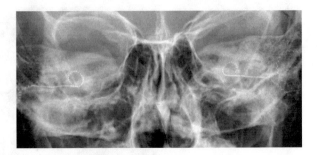

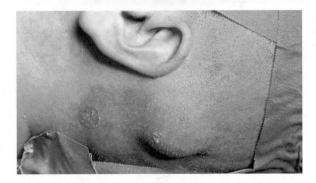

Fig. 10.9 Left side. The patient had a cochlear implantation 8 years and was using it regularly. They noticed a sudden swelling in the retroauricular region that corresponded to the position of the cochlear implant receiver. Although the patient was treated with antibiotics and the wound was revised, no significant improvement of the condition occurred. The surface of the implant had become covered with the bacterial biofilm. The inner part of the cochlear implant had to be explanted and was re-implanted once the infection was healed. Such complications occur rarely

Fig. 10.10 Ultrasound
image of bacterial biofilm
around the cochlear
implant receiver. The fluid
(white asterisk) covers the
implant body (orange
arrow) is related to the
presence of biofilm. Visible
above it is the skin with the
subcutaneous tissue
(orange asterisk)

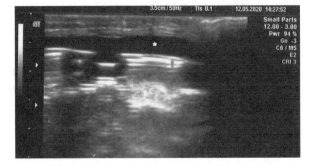

References

1. Almeida GFL, Martins MF, Costa LBAD, Costa OAD, Martinho de Carvalho AC. Sequential bilateral cochlear implant: results in children and adolescents. Braz J Otorhinolaryngol. 2019;85(6):774–9. https://doi.org/10.1016/j.bjorl.2018.07.008.
2. Manrique M, Ramos Á, de Paula Vernetta C, Gil-Carcedo E, Lassaletta L, Sanchez-Cuadrado I, Espinosa JM, Batuecas Á, Cenjor C, Lavilla MJ, Núñez F, Cavalle L, Huarte A. Guideline on cochlear implants. Acta Otorrinolaringol Esp (Engl Ed). 2019;70(1):47–54. https://doi.org/10.1016/j.otorri.2017.10.007.
3. Naples JG, Ruckenstein MJ. Cochlear implant. Otolaryngol Clin North Am. 2020;53(1):87–102.
4. Deep NL, Dowling EM, Jethanamest D, Carlson ML. Cochlear implantation: an overview. J Neurol Surg Skull Base. 2019;80(2):169–77.
5. Stöver T, Leinung M, Loth A. Which quality does make the difference in cochlear-implant therapy? Laryngorhinootologie. 2020;99(S 01):S107–64. https://doi.org/10.1055/a-1019-9381.
6. Goldfinger Y, Natan M, Sukenik CN, Banin E, Kronenberg J. Biofilm prevention on cochlear implants. Cochlear Implants Int. 2014;15(3):173–8.

Bone Conduction Devices

11

Implantable bone conduction devices (BCD) have developed in the last four decades. In general, a bone conduction transducer which is coupled percutaneously or transcutaneously to the skull and the vibrations are transmitted to the inner ear.

The bone-anchored hearing aid (BAHA) was the first system that was developed. The percutaneous device consists of a bone-anchored titanium implant, abutment, and a processor, which is attached to the abutment.

The transcutaneous device consists of a bone-anchored titanium implant, an internal magnet, an external magnet, and a processor (Fig. 11.1).

Percutaneous transmission is 10–15 dB more efficient than transcutaneous transmission.

Bone construction devices can also be active or adhered to the skin.

Indications for bone anchored-hearing aid are significant bilateral conductive or mixed hearing loss where middle ear surgery cannot bring any improvement and the patient is unable to wear conventional hearing aids. Audiological indications now include conductive and mixed hearing loss and single sided deafness (Fig. 11.2). Medical indications include radically operated patients with chronic otitis, external auditory canal atresia, patients who lost their hearing in vestibular schwannoma surgery and otosclerosis [1, 2] (Fig. 11.3).

Patients with profound unilateral sensorineural hearing loss or deafness have difficulty hearing in noisy situations, especially when speech is presented to the side with the hearing deficit. BAHA improves speech understanding in most environments with excessive background noise [3]. Satisfaction regarding the quality of sound and wearing comfort in patients with unilateral deafness was greater with percutaneous than with transcutaneous BAHA device [4].

The functional gain of bone conduction devices can be defined as the difference between aided sound-field thresholds and bone conduction thresholds. The maximum functional gain of the basic device is between 5 and 10 dB in the mid frequencies. The air-bone gap can be closed successfully, but any possible sensorineural hearing loss can only be partly compensated [2]. Also, the size of the air-bone gap

J. Rebol, *Otoscopy Findings*, https://doi.org/10.1007/978-3-031-03979-9_11

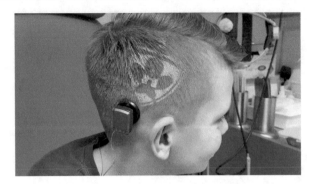

Fig. 11.1 A boy with a transcutaneous BCD. The patient was operated because of single sided deafness. In this system, the internal magnet is attached to the titanium implant and covered with skin. The external speech processor is attached to the external magnet. The hearing gain with devices in transcutaneous systems is lower than in percutaneous systems because of the loss of vibrations through the skin. It is important to place the device in children the soonest possible

Fig. 11.2 A pure-tone audiogram of a patient suitable for BAHA. Air conduction is at 80–90 dB, the air-bone gap is between 40 and 50 dB. The patient would not benefit from a conventional hearing aid as much as they would with a bone conduction device. Bone conduction levels, which should be within conversational speech frequencies between 30 and 50 dB, are important in deciding for a bone conduction device

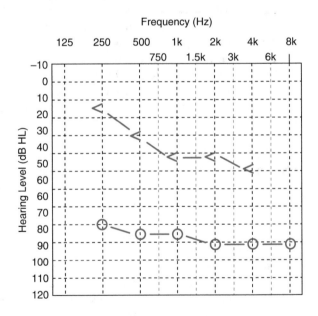

is important—if it exceeds about 25 dB, better audiometric results can be expected with bone conduction devices as with conventional hearing aids.

The advantage of BAHA is in no occlusion of the EAC. The EAC and the radical cavity can be normally ventilated after canal down mastoidectomy. The patient can also test the device before surgery, even for a longer period in different environments. Such testing improves the uptake of the device [5]. The surgical procedure is predictable and safe. In adults the procedure takes about 20–30 min under local anaesthesia. The surgical procedure is reversible and there is no risk of hearing loss following surgery.

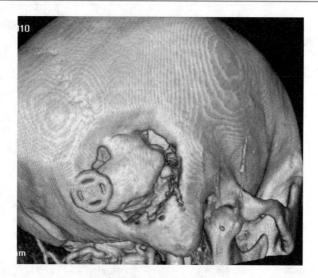

Fig. 11.3 A patient with single side deafness. The patient was operated through the suboccipital approach because of a vestibular schwannoma. The BCD transmits vibrations from the operated side to the contralateral cochlea. If the cochlear nerve is injured during the surgery, BCD is the only option for restoring hearing on the affected side. For better transmission of vibrations, it is important to place the titanium implant in the solid bone

Fig. 11.4 Right side. Surgery to fit a percutaneous bone conduction device (BCD). The titanium implant with an abutment is placed 5 cm posterosuperiorly to the EAC. The abutment is covered with hydroxyapatite in the lower part to reduce soft tissue reaction. In adults the operation is performed under local anaesthesia

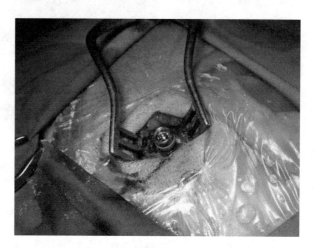

An incision is made about 5 cm posterosuperiorly of the EAC. A titanium implant is placed with low-speed torque setting under irrigation, which prevents the bone from overheating and later allows the implant to integrate into the bone. In percutaneous systems, an abutment is attached to the titanium implant (Figs. 11.4 and 11.5), in transcutaneous systems an internal magnet is attached. The processor is fitted about 3 weeks after the surgery.

The Holgers grading system of postoperative skin irritation is widely used for describing the state of the skin around the abutment in percutaneous systems. Grade

Fig. 11.5 The same patient as in Fig. 11.2. An opening is made in the skin for the abutment using the biopsy punch posteriorly of the incision

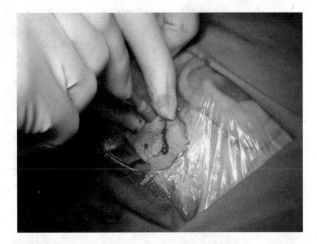

Fig. 11.6 The abutment for a percutaneous BCD. The skin around the abutment is without any inflammation and adheres around the abutment—Holgers grade 0

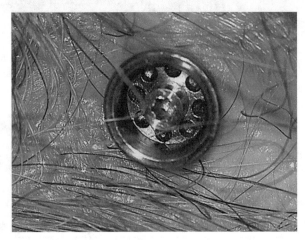

0 means no irritation; grade 1, slight redness; grade 2, red and moist tissue; grade 3, granulation tissue; and grade 4, infection and overgrowth of the skin over the abutment (Figs. 11.6, 11.7, 11.8, 11.9, and 11.10). Grades 1–2 can be treated with local therapy, grades 3–4 may require oral antibiotic therapy or even excision of the skin if overgrowth develops [6].

The most common skin problems in BAHA patients are local irritation and skin regrowth around the abutment. Comorbidities such as diabetes or dermatological and other systemic diseases certainly contribute to complication rates. Patients with a higher body mass index (BMI) also have significantly more skin problems than patients with a lower BMI.

The degree of soft tissue reactions observed in patients during follow-up can change over the years. After 2 years, the percentage of skin reactions decreases to below 10% [7].

Fig. 11.7 Left ear. The skin around the abutment is inflamed, red and moist inferiorly—Holgers grade 2. The condition is reversible. Local therapy with antibiotics and corticosteroid ointment is necessary

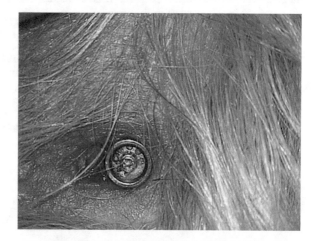

Fig. 11.8 Another patient with granulation tissue around the abutment—Holgers grade 3. Granulations can be excised and the skin treated with antibiotics and corticosteroid ointment

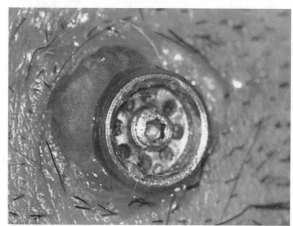

Fig. 11.9 Skin overgrowth. The skin is swollen and the abutment is already partially covered with skin—Holgers grade 4

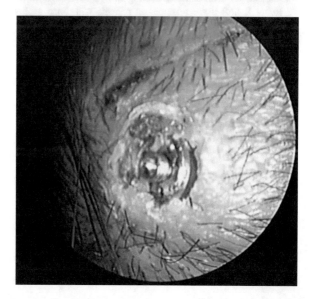

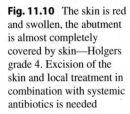

Fig. 11.10 The skin is red and swollen, the abutment is almost completely covered by skin—Holgers grade 4. Excision of the skin and local treatment in combination with systemic antibiotics is needed

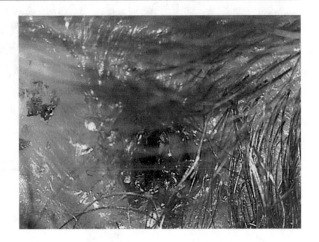

References

1. Tjoellstroem A, Hakansson B. The bone-anchored hearing aid. Otolaryngol Clin North Am. 1995;28:53–72.
2. Snik AF, Bosman AJ, Mylanus EA, Cremers CW. Candidacy for bone-anchored aid. Audiol Neurootol. 2004;9(4):190–6.
3. House JW, Kutz JW Jr, Chung J, Fisher LM. Bone-anchored hearing aid subjective benefit for unilateral deafness. Laryngoscope. 2010;120(3):601–7.
4. Svagan M, Povalej Brzan P, Rebol J. Comparison of satisfaction between patients using percutaneous and transcutaneous bone conduction devices. Otol Neurotol. 2019;40(5):651–7.
5. Powell R, Wearden A, Pardesi SM, Green K. Understanding the low uptake of bone-anchored hearing aids: a review. J Laryngol Otol. 2017;131(3):190–201.
6. Holgers KM, Tjellström A, Bjursten LM, Erlandson BE. Soft tissue reactions around percutaneous implants: a clinical study of soft tissue conditions around skin penetrating titanium implants for bone anchored hearing aids. Am J Otol. 1988;9(1):56–9.
7. Rebol J. Soft tissue reactions in patients with bone anchored hearing aids. Ir J Med Sci. 2015;184(2):487–91.

Postoperative Conditions 12

See Figs. 12.1, 12.2, 12.3, 12.4, 12.5, 12.6, 12.7, 12.8, and 12.9.

12.1 Tympanoplasty

Tympanoplasty is a procedure in which the disease in the middle ear is removed with or without the closure of the perforation. It can be also combined with a mastoidectomy. Otologists use the expression tympanoplasty mainly for closing the perforation of the eardrum. For the reconstruction we use perichondrium, taken

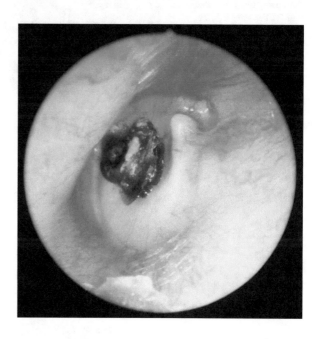

Fig. 12.1 Left ear. The tympanic tube (TT) is extruded. The TT is embedded in the crust on the surface of the eardrum and was removed with the fine forceps

J. Rebol, *Otoscopy Findings*, https://doi.org/10.1007/978-3-031-03979-9_12

Fig. 12.2 Right ear. Situation after a TT insertion, which has already been removed. There is a small retraction in the anteroinferior part of the eardrum and myringosclerosis, sequelae after TT insertion, can be observed

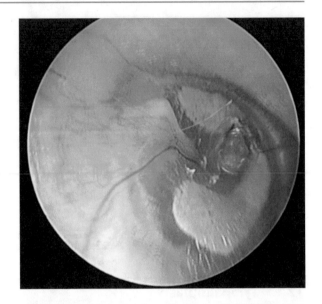

Fig. 12.3 Right ear. Patient with Samter's Triad or AERD (bronchial asthma, sensitivity to NSAIDs and nasal polyps). A myringotomy was made and a TT inserted. After the TT extrusion, a polypoid tissue began to appear from the myringotomy. Permanent suppurative secretion was also exuded through the perforation

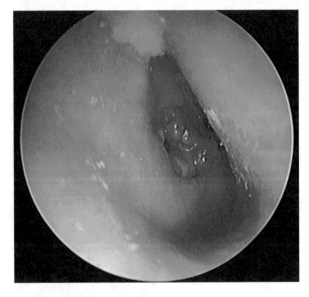

Fig. 12.4 Right ear. Another patient with Samter's Triad or AERD. After the insertion of the TT, the secretion dried in the TT lumen, blocking ventilation of the middle ear

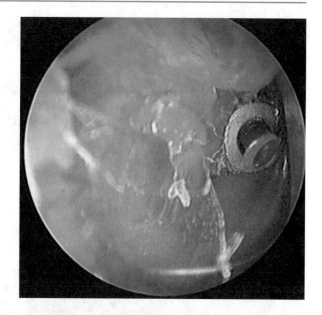

Fig. 12.5 Right ear. A 7-year-old girl presented with purulent discharge from the ear. The eardrum was covered with pus and granulation tissue was seen in the posteroinferior part of the eardrum. A TT previously was inserted in another country and the parents were told that the TTs were extruded. After cleaning the EAC, a metal wire could be identified on the surface of the eardrum

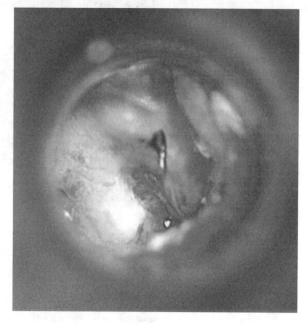

Fig. 12.6 Right ear. The same patient as in the previous figure. After raising of the tympanomeatal flap under general anaesthesia, a TT was discovered in the middle ear. The metal wire seen in the previous image was attached to the TT and protruded through the eardrum. Extrusion of TTs has to be properly documented in order to avoid accidentally retaining the foreign body in the middle ear

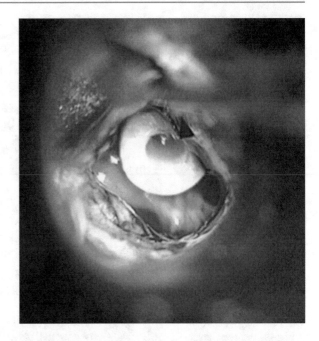

Fig. 12.7 Operation on exostoses in the right ear. The operation is performed through the retroauricular approach. The skin covering the exostoses is moved in a medial direction and covered with absorbent cotton. Exostoses are especially prominent on the anterior and posterior wall of the EAC

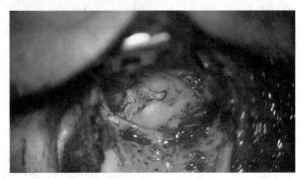

Fig. 12.8 The same patient as in the previous figure. The exostoses were drilled away with a diamond burr, the skin is repositioned and covers the medial part of the EAC. The skin is covered with two pieces of fluorosilicone rubber

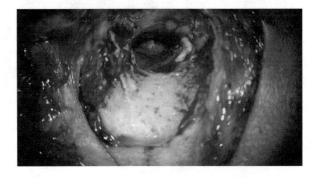

Fig. 12.9 Left ear. Dehiscence in the posterior wall of the EAC 2 weeks after the removal of exostoses. The skin covering the exostosis was very thin and had not healed. After 2 months the dehiscence healed spontaneously

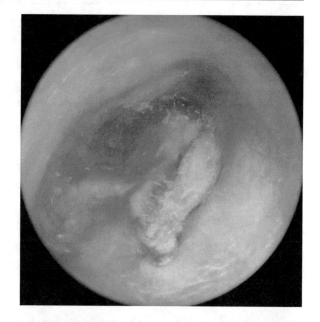

Fig. 12.10 Right ear. The patient had a small perforation in the anteroinferior quadrant of the eardrum. Under local anaesthesia a piece of fat was taken from the ear lobule, the edge of the perforation was removed, and fat was inserted into the perforation. The perforation healed and a yellow tissue can still be identified in the anteroinferior quadrant of the eardrum

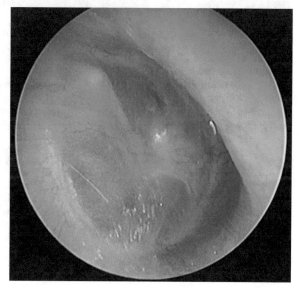

from the tragus or concha, or fascia of the temporal muscle. Cartilage in one piece or shaped and used as palisades is also very useful for reconstruction. Cartilage is very convenient for preventing the development of retractions of the eardrum and for covering titanium prostheses in ossiculoplasty (Figs. 12.10, 12.11, 12.12, 12.13, and 12.14).

Fig. 12.11 Left ear. Another patient after fat myringoplasty. The perforation was located close to the annulus between the anterosuperior and inferior ear quadrant

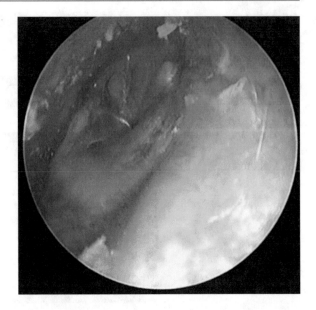

Fig. 12.12 Right ear. Situation after tympanoplasty in the inferior part of the eardrum. A slice of cartilage was inserted into the defect and covered with the perichondrium

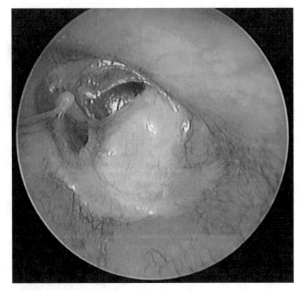

Ossiculoplasty is the reconstruction of the middle ear ossicular chain that has been disrupted or destroyed. Interpositioned devices are used to help regain the original mechanics of the ossicular chain and transfer sound energy to the inner ear.

It is often performed together with a tympanoplasty because perforations of the eardrum are often linked to ossicular chain defects.

Tympanoplasties were first classified by the German otologist Horst Ludwig Wullstein. Over the years various tympanoplasty classifications have been in use. We use a version of the Wullstein classification modified by Prof. Mirko Tos, who classified tympanoplasties according to the following types [1]:

Fig. 12.13 Left ear. Condition after tympanoplasty. The patient had a perforation in the posterior part of the eardrum. The defect was closed with cartilage and perichondrium. The perforation is closed, the eardrum is white because of the cartilage slice that had been put in place to prevent retraction

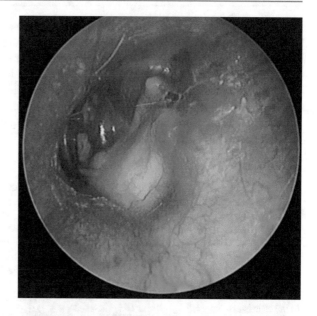

Fig. 12.14 Left ear. Condition after CWU mastoidectomy and scutumplasty (reconstruction of the lateral attic wall). In the posterior part of the eardrum is a cartilage slice which covers the partial ossicular prosthesis. Scutumplasty was also performed with a piece of cartilage. The eardrum in the anterior part is retracted due to Eustachian tube dysfunction

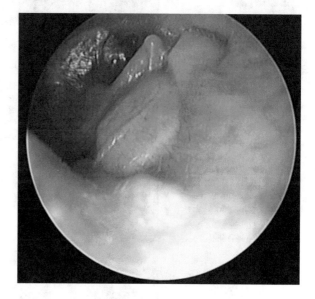

Tympanoplasty type 1 means reconstruction of the eardrum with an intact ossicular chain. Type 2 is a reconstruction when the long process of the incus is missing and the defect is reconstructed with a partial ossicular replacement prosthesis (PORP)—interposition. In type 3 the stapes suprastructure is also absent and the defect is reconstructed with a total ossicular replacement prosthesis (TORP)—columella. In type 4 the reconstructed eardrum is positioned onto the stapes footplate. In type 5a a fenestration of the lateral semicircular canal and in type 5b a platinectomy (removal of the stapes footplate) is performed.

For the reconstruction of the ossicular chain, the patient's own ossicles can be used (especially the incus) as well as prostheses made of titanium or hydroxyapatite, which are biocompatible. Titanium is a satisfactory material for use in ossicular reconstruction because of its ease of insertion, tissue tolerance, and low rate of extrusion.

Interposed prostheses transmit vibrations more effectively if placed parallel to the axis rather than at an angle. A large plate on the upper part of the prosthesis offers a slight acoustic advantage owing to the larger sound collecting area (Figs. 12.15, 12.16, 12.17, 12.18, 12.19, 12.20, 12.21, 12.22, 12.23, 12.24, 12.25, and 12.26) [2].

Fig. 12.15 Left ear. Condition after ossiculoplasty and scutumplasty. A hydroxyapatite (HA) total ossicular replacement prosthesis (TORP) is positioned under the malleus handle, the defect in the attic is also covered with a HA plate

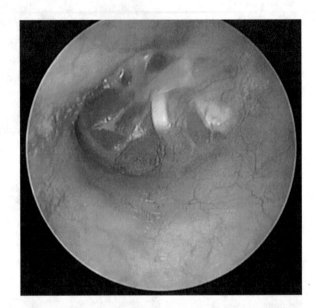

Fig. 12.16 Right ear. A Goldenberg TORP placed under the eardrum in the posteroinferior part of the eardrum. The rest of the eardrum is sclerotic

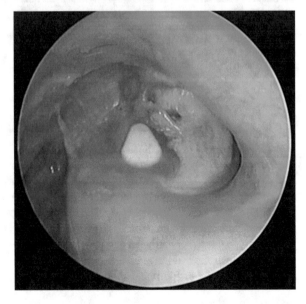

Fig. 12.17 Left ear. Condition after ossiculoplasy with the patient's own incus as an interposition graft. The short process of the incus is placed under the malleus handle

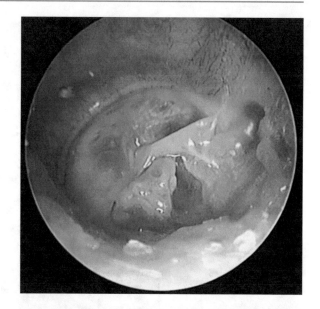

Fig. 12.18 Right ear. During the operation the tympanomeatal flap was raised and the ossicular chain can be assessed. The long process of the incus is missing, but the stapes suprastructure is intact. The defect was corrected with a PORP placed on the head of stapes

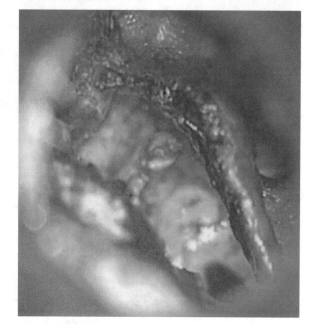

Fig. 12.19 Right ear. Condition after ossiculoplasty where a HA PORP was placed on the head of stapes and under the handle of malleus

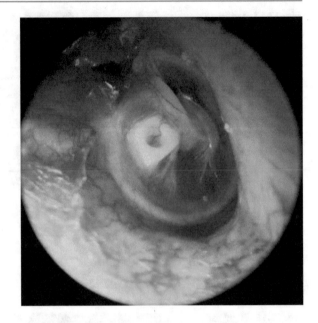

Fig. 12.20 The incus removed after fixation in the attic. On the top of the incus body is the bony tissue by which the ossicle was fixed to the attic roof. During the operation, the incus was replaced by a PORP

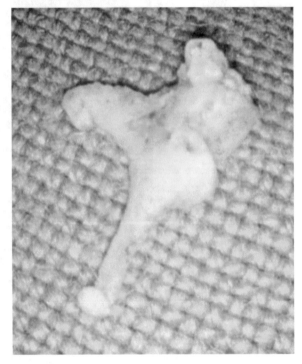

Fig. 12.21 Right ear. The posterior part of the eardrum is positioned anteriorly. In the middle ear a defect of the long process of the incus and the stapes suprastructure can be identified. The stapes footplate is intact

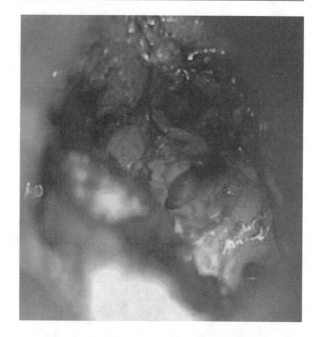

Fig. 12.22 The same ear as in the previous figure. A Goldenberg TORP was placed on the stapes footplate. Part of the prosthesis can be seen under the tympanomeatal flap

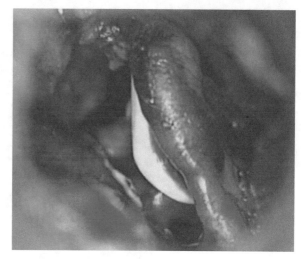

Fig. 12.23 The same
patient as in the previous
two figures. In the next
stage a slice of cartilage
was placed on top of the
TORP. The tympanomeatal
flap is temporarily moved
towards the handle of
malleus

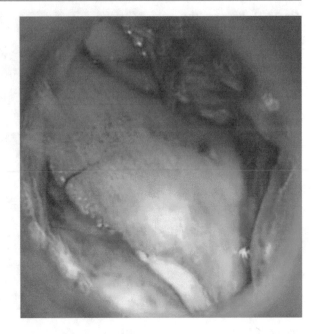

Fig. 12.24 The last stage
of the operation from the
previous three figures. The
cartilage slice is covered
with the perichondrium
and the tympanomeatal
flap is repositioned in its
original position

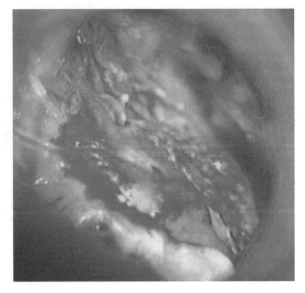

Fig. 12.25 Right ear. Condition after ossiculoplasty with a HA TORP. Because of the cholesteatoma, the long process of the incus and the stapes suprastructure were resorbed. The prosthesis is put on the stapes footplate and under the handle of malleus. The eardrum is positioned normally. The patient's hearing is almost normal because of good sound transmission

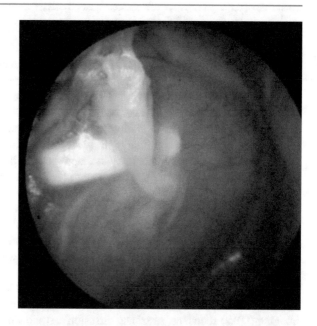

Fig. 12.26 Left ear. Situation after the removal of a cholesteatoma by performing a CWD mastoidectomy. The incus and stapes suprastructure defect was corrected with a Wehrs HA TORP. After a CWD mastoidectomy, the volume of the middle ear is usually reduced ("flat eardrum") and the hearing results after a CWD mastoidectomy are worse when compared with CWU mastoidectomy. Over time the eardrum retracted and the prosthesis is partially extruded. Because the air-bone gap in this patient was moderate, the prosthesis was left in place

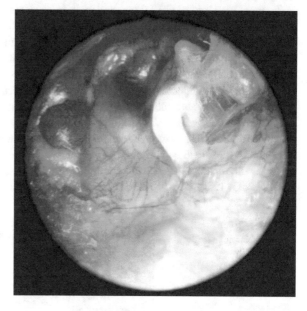

12.2   Cholesteatoma Surgery

In atticotomy, the lateral wall of the attic (scutum) is removed and the area lateral to malleus head and incus body is exposed. At mastoidectomy, the mastoid cells are removed to expose and remove any cholesteatomatous tissue. In canal wall up (CWU) mastoidectomy, the posterior EAC wall as well as the normal anatomy of the ear are preserved. The operation is usually combined with a posterior tympanotomy, tympanoplasty, and scutumplasty (reconstruction of the lateral attic wall). Advantages of CWU mastoidectomy are rapid healing time, easier long-term care, hearing aids are easier to fit, and less water precautions are needed. The disadvantages are that it is technically a more difficult procedure than CWD mastoidectomy, a staged operation is often necessary, recurrent disease is possible, and any residual disease is harder to detect. Patients are suitable for the CWU mastoidectomy, if they have normal mastoid pneumatisation, normal tubal function, if the cholesteatoma is limited to the mastoid without destruction of the EAC wall, and if they are able to attend the "second look" operation [3].

Patients operated with CWU mastoidectomy are told to come for regular follow-ups. Cholesteatoma can be also followed with MRI where, with diffusion weighted imaging (DWI) sequence, restricted diffusion can show the presence of the disease.

In canal wall down (CWD) mastoidectomy (open technique), the posterior wall of the EAC is removed. The middle ear is reconstructed. The operation is indicated in patients with the poor pneumatisation of the mastoid, tubal dysfunction, in elderly patients, and patients with poor compliance. A CWD mastoidectomy is performed in extensive cholesteatoma, labyrinth fistula, and recurrent cholesteatoma.

In radical mastoidectomy no middle ear and eardrum reconstruction is performed, the Eustachian tube is also obliterated. Meatoplasty is also an important part of the operation in CWD mastoidectomy and radical mastoidectomy when the entrance to the EAC has to be widened. Parts of the concha cartilage are excised to get a wide exposure and ventilation of the cavity. The cleaning of the cavity is much easier, if the meatoplasty is wide enough (Figs. 12.27, 12.28, 12.29, 12.30, 12.31, 12.32, 12.33, 12.34, 12.35, 12.36, 12.37, 12.38, 12.39, 12.40, and 12.41).

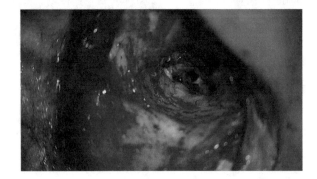

Fig. 12.27 Right ear. The retroauricular approach in a patient with cholesteatoma. The skin of the EAC as well as the tympanomeatal flap are moved out of the way. The cholesteatoma is the white mass that can be identified in the attic

Fig. 12.28 Right ear. Continuation of the operation in patient from the previous figure. A CWU mastoidectomy was performed. The tip of the aspirator is pointing towards the cholesteatoma sac in the antrum of the mastoid

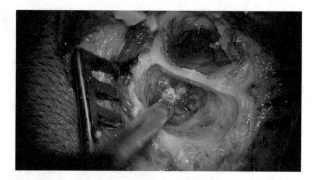

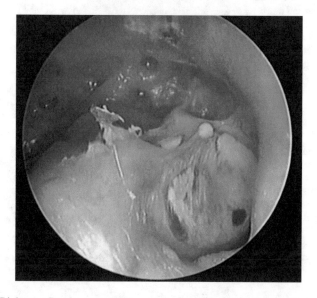

Fig. 12.29 Right ear. Bondy operation is a type of modified radical mastoidectomy, where a CWD mastoidectomy is performed without disturbing the ossicular chain. The operation can be performed in cases of attic cholesteatoma extending to the mastoid. The operation can preserve good preoperative hearing. In this patient the eardrum is sclerotic but positioned normally, the volume of the middle ear is normal and the patient's hearing is almost normal. Patients require regular cleaning of the cavity and have to be careful with water exposure

Fig. 12.30 Left ear. The patient had an extensive cholesteatoma and a CWD mastoidectomy was performed. The posterior EAC wall and the mastoid cells were drilled away and the mastoid cavity was connected with the EAC. The cavity is dry and clean. The eardrum is retracted especially in the anterior part. In such cases cavity cerumen and crusts can accumulate and periodic (yearly) cleaning is recommended

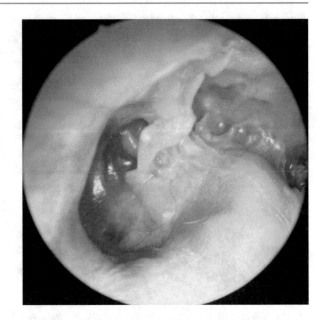

Fig. 12.31 Left ear. Condition after a CWD mastoidectomy. Cerumen and some crusts have accumulated in the mastoid cavity and need to be cleaned

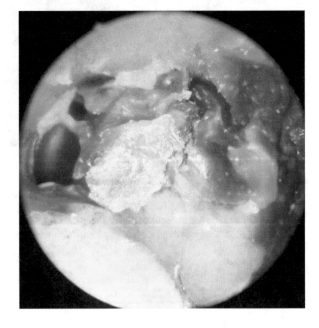

Fig. 12.32 Right ear. Condition after a CWD mastoidectomy. The mastoid cavity is dry and clean. The eardrum is retracted, with no perforation. A cholesteatoma pearl can be identified in the anterior attic wall. This is easily removed at the office and needs to be attended to because of possibility of growing

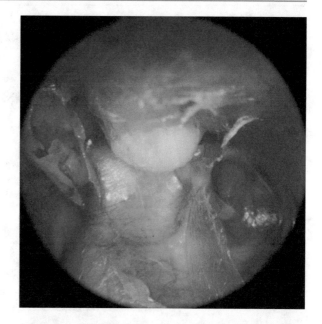

Fig. 12.33 Right ear. Condition after a CWD mastoidectomy. The cavity is dry and clean. Five small cholesteatoma pearls can be seen on the roof of the attic

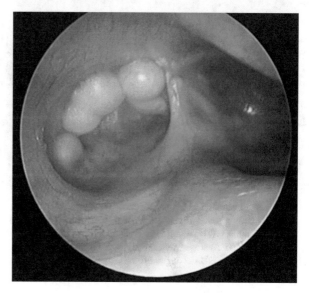

Fig. 12.34 Right ear. Condition after a radical mastoidectomy. The patient was operated on 50 years ago. After cleaning and aspirating the cavity, the patient always had severe vertigo and nausea. The arrows mark the cause of the problems—a fistula in the lateral semicircular canal

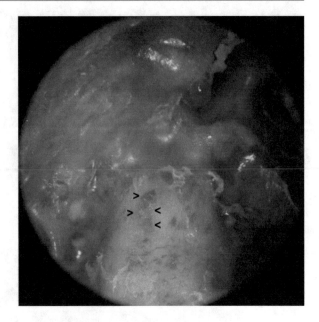

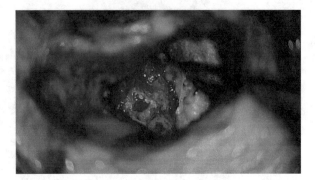

Fig. 12.35 Left ear. The image was taken during a cholesteatoma operation. Prior to the operation the patient complained of vertigo. A high-resolution CT scan revealed a fistula in the lateral semicircular canal. A CWU mastoidectomy was performed. The matrix of the cholesteatoma was raised and removed. The fistula was immediately covered with the temporal fascia. The patient's bone conduction remained unchanged after the operation

Fig. 12.36 Left ear. A
CWD mastoidectomy was
performed on the patient.
The entire cavity is wet,
covered with a thin layer of
pus. Granulation tissue can
be seen in the medial part
of the EAC, coming from
the middle ear mucosa.
The tissue has to be
removed and the cavity
treated with local
antibiotics or antiseptics

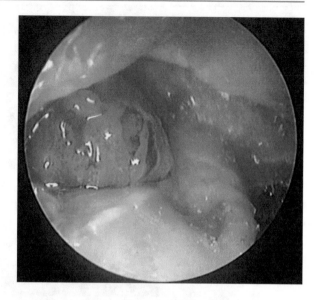

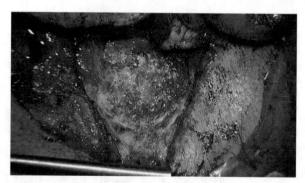

Fig. 12.37 Left ear. The patient was operated because of a cholesteatoma many years ago. A
modified radical mastoidectomy was performed. They suffered from constant discharge from the
cavity, which could not be cured with local therapy. The picture was taken during the operation in
which the cavity was obliterated with the bioactive glass and the posterior EAC wall was reconstructed with cartilage. In the picture the mastoid cavity is filled with the bioactive glass and will
be covered with the periosteal flap

Fig. 12.38 Left ear. Condition after the mastoid obliteration with bioactive glass and the EAC posterior wall reconstruction. The EAC is dry, the diameter of the EAC is normal and the eardrum is also intact. The patient has no problems with chronic discharge

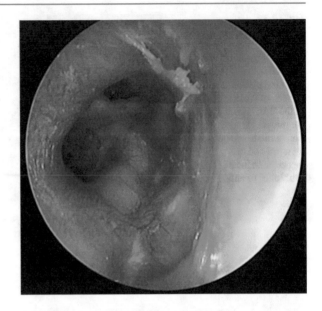

Fig. 12.39 Left ear. The patient had a cholesteatoma operation. CWU mastoidectomy, tympanoplasty, and scutumplasty were performed. The eardrum is slightly retracted, opaque, and a small cholesteatoma pearl can be seen on the handle of malleus. The defect in the attic was reconstructed with a cartilage graft. A small cholesteatoma pearl can also be seen on the superior wall of the EAC lateral to the scutumplasty

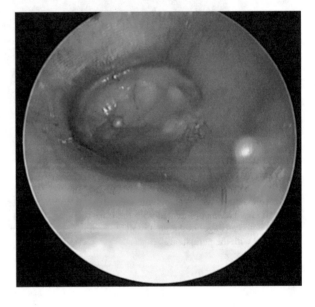

Fig. 12.40 Left ear.
Condition after the CWU
mastoidectomy,
tympanoplasty, and
scutumplasty. The
posterior part of the
eardrum is white because a
cartilage slice was
positioned there to cover
the titanium PORP. The
rest of the eardrum is
transparent. The attic
defect was reconstructed
with a HA plate

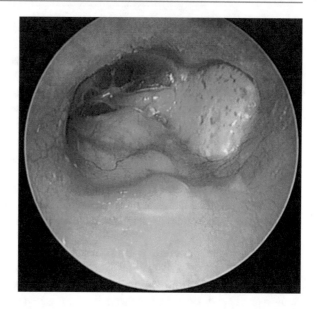

Fig. 12.41 Left ear.
Another patient after a
CWU mastoidectomy,
tympanoplasty, and
scutumplasty. The defect in
the attic was reconstructed
with the cortical bone,
cartilage, and
perichondrium were used
for the tympanoplasty.
There is a sclerotic plaque
in the anterior upper
quadrant of the eardrum
and a small retraction
pocket in the inferior
quadrants

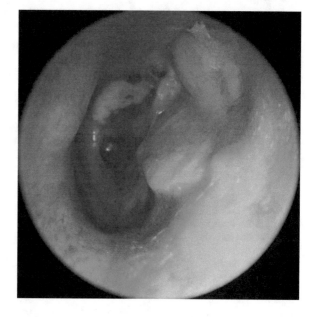

12.3   Surgical Management of Otosclerosis

The term *otosclerosis* was introduced by Politzer in 1894 and refers to the final stage of the disease where the bone is sclerotic and hardened. Otosclerosis is a localised disease of the bone derived from the otic capsule and characterised by alternating phases of bone resorption and formation. Histopathologically the otosclerotic process is characterised by an abnormal bone remodelling, resulting in replacement of otic capsule bone with a hypercellular woven bone, which may undergo further remodelling to eventually reach a mosaic sclerotic appearance. The disease is found only in humans and is limited to the temporal bone.

The site of predilection is the fissula ante fenestram which lies anterior of the stapes footplate. The cause of otosclerosis can be hereditary, infection with paramyxoviruses, and hormones may also play an important role in worsening of the disease.

Otoscopic status in otosclerosis is normal. The Schwartze sign is a diagnostic indicator in the active phase of otosclerosis—increased vascularity on the promontory can be observed through the eardrum. Diagnosis is set by audiometry that shows conductive or mixed hearing loss, as well as tympanometry and stapedial reflex.

Surgery is considered for patients with conductive hearing loss of at least 15 dB in frequencies 250–1000 Hz or higher. A typical finding in otosclerosis is also the Carhart notch which means a depression in bone conduction at 2000 Hz. A Rinne test should also be negative with a 512 Hz fork.

If both sides are affected with otosclerosis, the ear with poorer hearing should be operated on first. After a successful operation of the first ear, the other ear may be operated after a period of around a year.

At stapedotomy, the stapes suprastructure is removed, a small opening in the stapes footplate is made and a prosthesis inserted, which is fixed to the long process of the incus. The results of these operations are very good (Figs. 12.42, 12.43, 12.44, and 12.45) [4, 5].

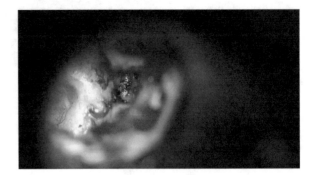

Fig. 12.42 Left ear. Operation on otosclerosis with an argon laser. The focus is on the stapes footplate, the stapes suprastructure was removed before. A rosette was created with the laser on the surface of the footplate. A stapedotomy will be performed at that point and a stapes prosthesis inserted

Fig. 12.43 Right ear. The final stage of the stapedotomy. The prosthesis was inserted into the stapedotomy and fixed with the laser onto the long process of the incus. The chorda tympani nerve is moved superiorly to get the access to the long process of the incus

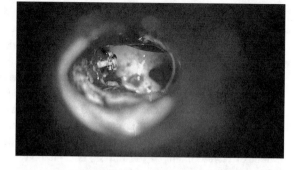

Fig. 12.44 Left ear. Condition after the stapedotomy. The eardrum is transparent. The prosthesis fixed onto the long process of the incus can be seen through the eardrum (arrow)

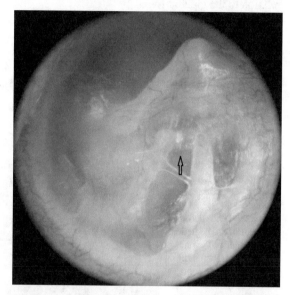

Fig. 12.45 Left ear. Otosclerosis may be combined with epitympanic fixation of the incus. In such cases the incus has to be removed and the prosthesis is inserted into the stapedotomy and fixed to the handle of malleus (arrow). Such an operation can be done also in cases of long process of the incus necrosis, in revision stapedotomy, or in operations of congenital malformations of the ossicular chain

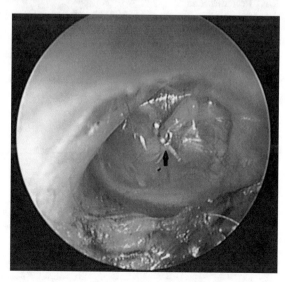

12.4 EAC Atresia

Deficiencies in the formation of the EAC is always connected with malformations of the ear. Congenital aural atresia is present in about one in 10,000–20,000 births and can also appear when various other syndromes are present. Unilateral atresia is more common than bilateral. Atresia of the EAC is also combined with malformations of the ossicular chain. The middle ear condition (development of the ossicular chain) and pneumatisation of the mastoid are often connected with the level of development of the auricle [6]. Preoperatively a CT scan is needed to establish the extent of development of the middle ear, pneumatisation of the mastoid, and the relation to the glenoid fossa.

The EAC atresia operation is usually corried out between the ages of 8 and 10 because by then the auricle has reached normal size. Surgery is performed with facial nerve monitoring because of the abnormal course of the nerve. After the operation the chance of restenosis of the EAC is high. Sometimes the surgery is not possible due to unfavourable middle ear conditions. Many patients also still need a hearing aid after the operation. A popular solution for these patients are bone-anchored hearing aids—BAHA (Figs. 12.46, 12.47, 12.48, and 12.49) (Chap. 11).

Fig. 12.46 Right ear. Condition after EAC reconstruction due to congenital atresia. Microtia can be seen with deformity of the auricle. The patient had conductive hearing loss. The entrance in the EAC is now open with some crusts inside the EAC. Reconstruction of the auricle can be performed in a separate operation

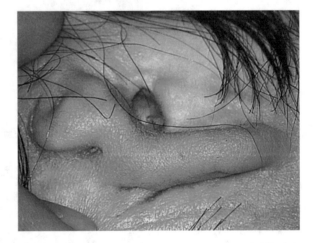

Fig. 12.47 Left ear. Beginning of the operation in congenital atresia of the EAC. The bony atretic plate can be seen without any lumen of the EAC

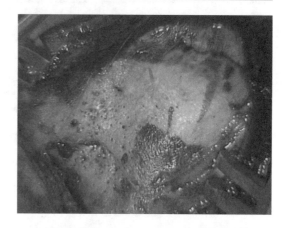

Fig. 12.48 The same ear as in the previous figure. A new EAC is drilled with the middle ear seen medially. In a small area the dura of the middle fossa is exposed and can be used for orientation when drilling the ear canal

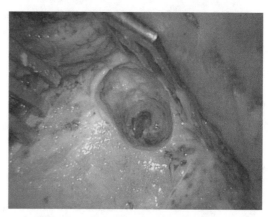

Fig. 12.49 Right ear. A small defect can be observed on the anterior wall of the EAC (white arrow). It caused saliva to enter the EAC during meals. Salivary fistulas of the parotid gland to the EAC are very rare. They develop after injury of the parenchyma or the gland ductus and also after surgery in the head and neck region. In this patient otosialorrhoea developed after parotid injury. It closed spontaneously

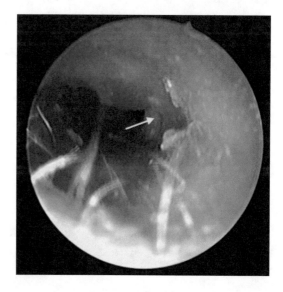

References

1. Tos M. Tympanoplasty—general. In: Tos M, editor. Manual of middle ear surgery, vol. 1. Stuttgart: Thieme; 1993. p. 238–44.
2. Dost P, Jahnke K. Biomaterials in reconstructive middle ear surgery. In: Jahnke K, editor. Middle ear surgery. New York: Thieme; 2004. p. 53–70.
3. Tos M. Classic intact canal wall mastoidectomy. In: Tos M, editor. Manual of middle ear surgery, vol. 2. New York: Thieme; 1995. p. 106–55.
4. Tos M. Otosclerosis. In: Surgical solutions for conductive hearing loss. New York: Thieme; 2000. p. 83–94.
5. Rebol J. Otosclerosis. In: Kountakis SE, editor. Encyclopedia of otolaryngology, head and neck surgery. Berlin: Springer; 2013. https://doi.org/10.1007/978-3-642-23499-6_702.
6. Tos M. Congenital atresia. In: Tos M, editor. Manual of middle ear surgery, vol. 3. New York: Thieme; 1997. p. 247–66.

Imaging of the Temporal Bone

13

Imaging of the temporal bone pathology is accomplished mainly by computed tomography (CT) and magnetic resonance imaging (MRI).

CT scans offers better spatial resolution compared to MRIs and allows good delineation of calcifications, cortical bone, air, and fat. MRI enables multiplanar imaging and provides better detail on soft tissue abnormalities. In the majority of cases one modality is the procedure of choice over the other. Imaging time in MRI is much longer and requires good patient cooperation to get high quality images. In small children as well as in patients with claustrophobia general anaesthesia is sometimes required [1, 2].

MRI is contraindicated in some patients with implanted metallic foreign bodies or metallic devices. In otology such devices are cochlear implant and active middle ear implants. Radiologists and technologists operating the MRI system should be informed by the patients about any devices and determine whether the patient can be exposed to the magnetic field without risk. Patients with stapedotomy and ossiculoplasty also have titanium prostheses in their middle ear. After the operation the patients are given documentation with an outline of instructions about exposure to MRI. Modern cochlear implants enable the exposition to the magnetic field of up to 3 T with a bandage around the head, but certain older-generation implants allow exposure of only up to 1.5 T, with some devices not allow any exposure at all. In such cases the magnet in the implant body can be temporarily removed for the duration of the investigation. The devices are produced by different companies and checking the manufacturer's instructions is very important. Patients with implanted middle ear titanium prostheses can normally be exposed to the magnetic field with these prostheses (Figs. 13.1, 13.2, 13.3, 13.4, 13.5, 13.6, 13.7, 13.8, 13.9, 13.10, 13.11, 13.12, 13.13, 13.14, 13.15, 13.16, 13.17, 13.18, 13.19, 13.20, 13.21, 13.22, 13.23, 13.24, 13.25, 13.26, 13.27, 13.28, 13.29, 13.30, 13.31, 13.32, and 13.33).

J. Rebol, *Otoscopy Findings*, https://doi.org/10.1007/978-3-031-03979-9_13

Fig. 13.1 CT scan in axial plane at the level of the epitympanum: 1—head of the malleus, 2—body of the incus, 3—short process of the incus, 4—mastoid antrum, 5—facial nerve, 6—cochlea, 7—vestibule

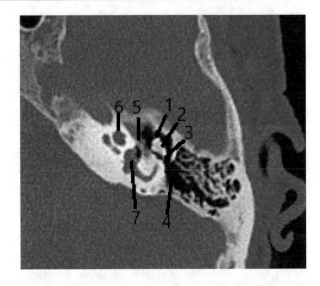

Fig. 13.2 CT scan in axial plane at the level of the mesotympanum: 1—handle of the malleus, 2—sinus tympani, 3—facial nerve, 4—round window niche, 5—basal turn of the cochlea, 6—carotid artery

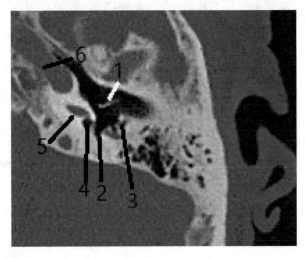

Fig. 13.3 CT scan in axial plane at the level of the EAC: 1- pinna, 2- the EAC, 3-glenoid fossa, 4- mastoid cells, 5- tympanic membrane, 6- tympanic cavity, 7- Eustachian tube, 8- carotid artery, 9- jugular foramen

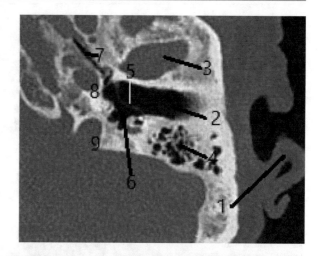

Fig. 13.4 CT scan in axial plane: on the right side, the condyle of the mandible is fractured and rotated. The anterior EAC bony wall is also fractured and the bone fragment is dislocated into the lumen of the EAC

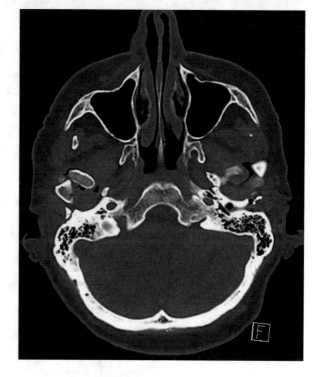

Fig. 13.5 The same patient as in the previous figure. A 3D CT reconstruction: the head of mandible is fractured and the bony fragment of the EAC is obstructing the lumen

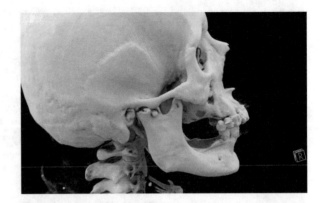

Fig. 13.6 CT scan in axial plane. Patient with necrotizing external otitis. The anterior wall of the left EAC is almost entirely resorbed (white arrow)

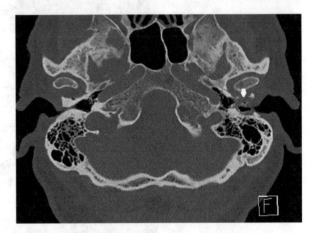

Fig. 13.7 Axial CT scan showing a longitudinal fracture in the left mastoid (orange arrow)

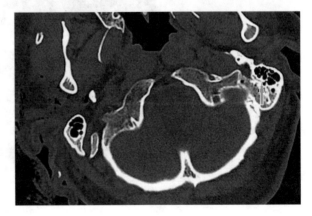

Fig. 13.8 A 3D CT reconstruction. An elliptical fracture of the squama of the temporal bone can be seen

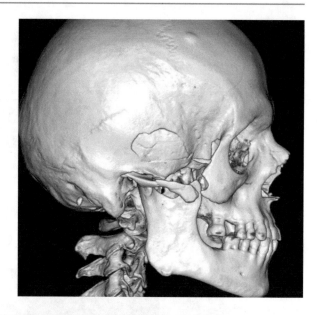

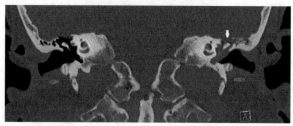

Fig. 13.9 CT scan in coronal plane. The patient had conductive hearing loss due to the presence of fluid in the middle ear. A TT was inserted. The patient had constant otorrhea from the operated ear. When asked about the background to the injury the patient remembered a fall some 50 years ago during when they were unconscious for a short time. The CT scan shows a defect in the middle fossa dura following the fracture of the temporal bone (white arrow). The discharge in the middle ear was cerebrospinal fluid (CSF), which flowed constantly through the fistula. The patient never got meningitis in the past 50 years

Fig. 13.10 CT scan in coronal plane: attic cholesteatoma on the left side with a defect of the scutum (lateral attic wall) (orange arrow). The cholesteatoma is spreading into the mastoid, ossicles in the attic are resorbed

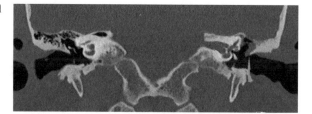

Fig. 13.11 CT scan in axial plane. The same patient as in the previous figure. On the left side a cholesteatoma can be detected in the mastoid. A fistula in the lateral semicircular canal can be seen. Before surgery the patient had problems with vertigo

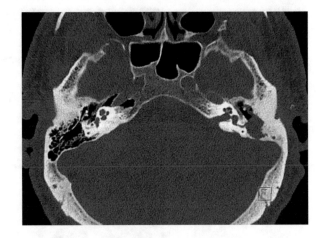

Fig. 13.12 T2 weighted MRI in coronal plane. The sequence renders fluids bright, while all other structures are dark. The structures that are inside fluid-filled spaces can be assessed easily regarding size and contour. On the right side, fluid surrounds the cholesteatoma in the mastoid. The contralateral side is dark because the mastoid cells are filled with air

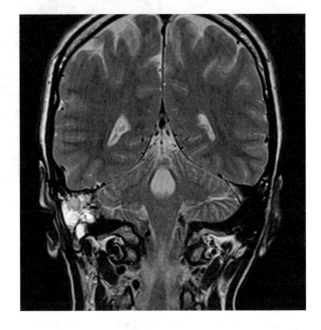

Fig. 13.13 The same patient as in the previous figure. Coronal DWI shows the lesion with restricted diffusion. High signal intensity is diagnostic for cholesteatoma. Such imaging can be used in follow-ups after a cholesteatoma operation

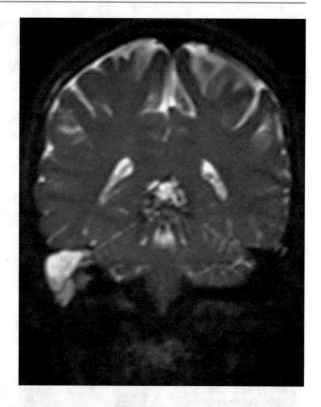

Fig. 13.14 CT scan in axial plane. The patient was operated on cholesteatoma in the left ear. After a CWD mastoidectomy, the patient often complained about chronic otorrhea from the operated ear. On the left side there is bioactive glass filling the mastoid

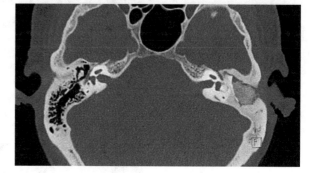

Fig. 13.15 Sigmoid sinus thrombosis left. There is a defect of contrast on the left (black arrow) and the sigmoid sinus on the right has normal contrast opacification (white arrow). The patient had chronic otitis on the left side

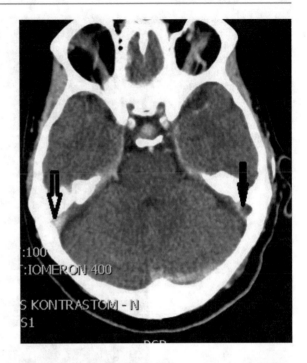

Fig. 13.16 CT scan with contrast, coronal plane. The same patient as shown in the previous figure. The sigmoid sinus thrombosis had also spread to the internal jugular vein in the neck (black arrow), where the contrast is not passing through the vein

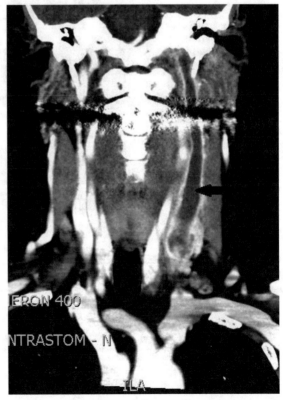

Fig. 13.17 Bezold abscess on the right side (asterisk). The coronal CT image shows an abscess (asterisk) inferior to the mastoid apex

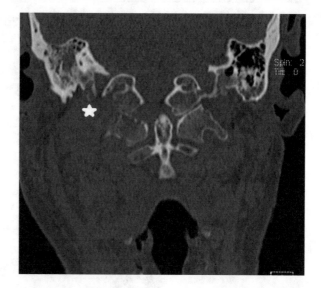

Fig. 13.18 CT scan in axial plane. A complication from mastoiditis on the right side with a spread of the infection through the apex of the mastoid to the soft tissues, forming an abscess called a Bezold's abscess (white asterisk)

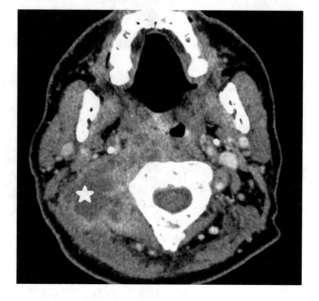

Fig. 13.19 Another complication of acute mastoiditis on the left side. After otitis the elderly patient had headache and ataxia. The CT scan in axial plane shows the abscess in the left cerebellar hemisphere (arrow)

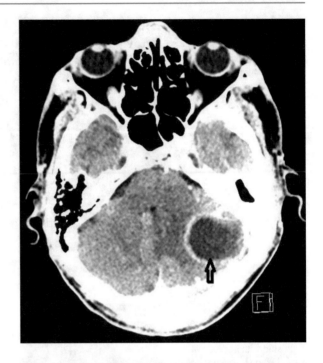

Fig. 13.20 CT scan in coronal plane. On the right the medial part of the EAC and the entire middle ear are filled with the tumour, which also erodes the bone at the tegmen tympani and at the level of hypotympanic cells (arrow)

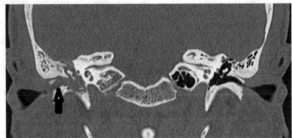

Fig. 13.21 CT scan in coronal plane. A 2-year-old child with bilateral destruction of the mastoid bone. Clinically otorrhea with swollen skin in the EAC was present. Biopsies were taken from both ears and revealed histiocytosis X

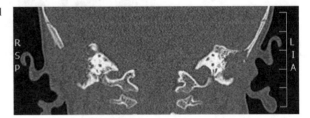

Fig. 13.22 CT scan in coronal plane. On the left side a bony destruction involving the temporomandibular joint and extending to the temporal bone can be observed

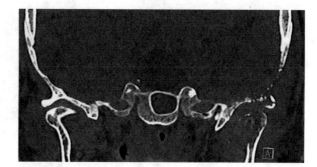

Fig. 13.23 A 3D CT reconstruction. The same patient as in the previous figure. A large defect in the temporal bone extending to the infratemporal fossa and temporomandibular joint can be seen on the patient's left side. The imaging was performed due to a CSF leak from the EAC. The osteolytic lesion was a metastasis from a uterine carcinoma

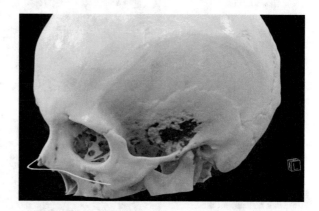

Fig. 13.24 Axial CT image. Abnormal calcifications in the basal turn of the cochlea (arrow) that are compatible with labyrinthitis ossificans. The patient suffered from meningitis in his boyhood and was a candidate for cochlear implantation

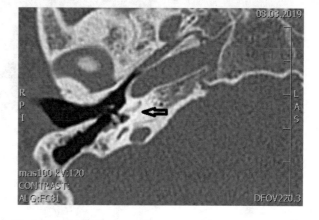

Fig. 13.25 Coronal CT image shows a tumour in the middle ear on the right side (orange arrow). Clinically a red mass was observed behind the intact eardrum, which was pulsating. On the image the tumour is located only in the middle ear without extension to the jugular foramen. These findings indicate a glomus tympanicum tumour

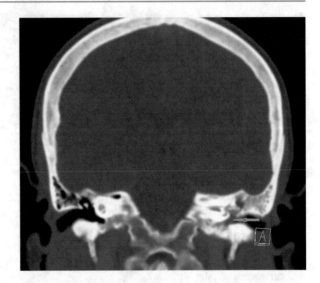

Fig. 13.26 The same patient as in the previous figure. An MRI scan in axial plane. The tumour in the middle ear, which extends into the Eustachian tube can be seen on the left side (orange arrow)

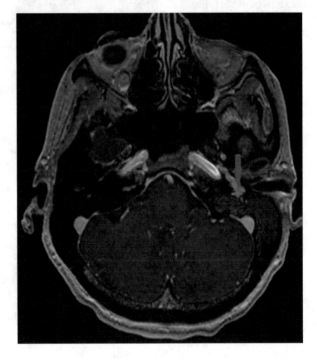

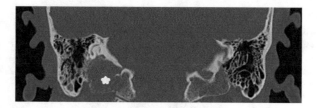

Fig. 13.27 Coronal bone algorithm CT. On the right side a large expansive lesion with bone erosion originating from the jugular foramen can be seen (asterisk). The finding is consistent with jugular paraganglioma

Fig. 13.28 Axial contrast-enhanced MRI T1 weighted image. The same patient as in the previous figure. On the right side is a tumour (orange arrow) in the jugular foramen with internal flow voids, which gives the lesion a typical "salt and pepper" appearance, characteristic of jugular paraganglioma

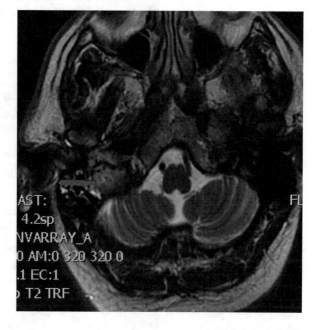

Fig. 13.29 Coronal
angio-MRI in the patient
with a jugular
paraganglioma on the left
side. The tumour is very
vascularised. Before
surgery embolisation is
performed by the
radiologist

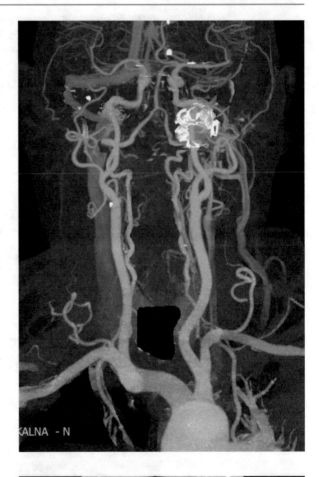

Fig. 13.30 Carotid
angiogram in the patient
before embolisation for a
jugular paraganglioma on
the right side. The patient
has an aplastic transverse
and sigmoid sinus on the
right. The sigmoid sinus is
usually closed during the
operation. In this case,
however, closure of the
sigmoid sinus would
severely compromise
intracranial venous
blood flow

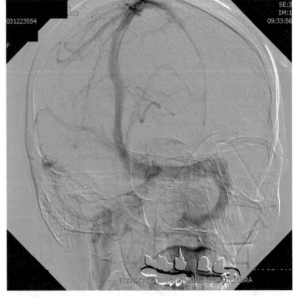

Fig. 13.31 Axial MRI with contrast T1 weighted. On the left side a tumour (most probably a vestibular schwannoma) extends from the internal auditory canal into the cerebellopontine angle with almost no impression on the brain stem (arrow)

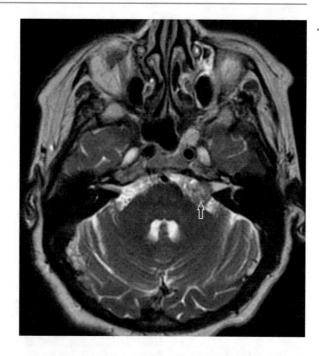

Fig. 13.32 X-ray after bilateral cochlear implantation, lateral view. The implant body is marked with the orange arrow, the magnet with the green arrow. Based on the shape of the body of the implant the radiologist can determine the series to which is belongs. The shape of the magnet suggests that it is a type that can be exposed to a magnetic field up to 1.5 T with a bandage around the head

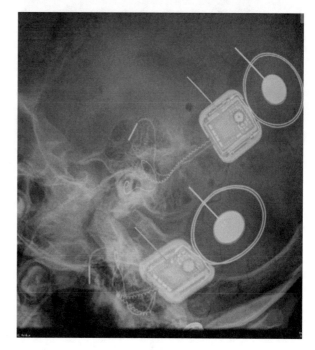

Fig. 13.33 X-ray, lateral view, after a unilateral cochlear implantation. The orange arrow marks the implant body of the latest generation of cochlear implants. The green arrow points to the magnet, which can turn when exposed to a magnetic field. A patient with this kind of device can be exposed to a magnetic field up to 3 T with a bandage around the head

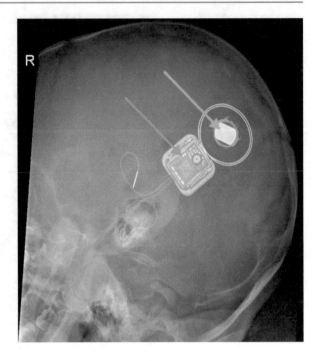

References

1. Juliano AF. Cross sectional imaging of the ear and temporal bone. Head Neck Pathol. 2018;12(3):302–20.
2. Cornelius RS. Temporal bone imaging. In: Hughes H, Pensak M, editors. Clinical otology. 3rd ed. New York: Thieme; 2007. p. 95–108.